STAY CONNECTED
It's My Hair! Magazine
www.itsmyhairmagazine.com
info@itsmyhairmagazine.com
Social Media: @itsmyhairmag

THE LITTLE SQUAD
BEHIND VOLUME 01
Ariel Johnson, Writer
Brianna Barnard, Researcher
Maria Aiam Angeles, Graphic Designer
Selena Milbry, Founder & Editor
CR142 Photos
LASEWOD Photography

DIRECTORY

BEAUTY FEATURE FROM LONDON, UNITED KINGDOM
MEET **DEBORAH FALCONER,** *MAKEUP ARTIST*

DIGITAL INFLUENCER
4 – 21
Discusses the start
of social media
in the 90's and
showcases several
influencers from
all around the world
on hair, beauty
and style.

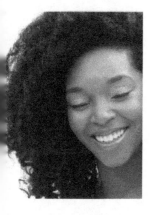

FRO COLLECTION
22 – 29
A little history on Afro's
plus innovative ways to
wear one.

COVER GIRL
30 – 39
Meet our cover girl
SHEILA NDINDA as
she talks hair, beauty,
favorite brands,
traveling and more.

COLOR COLLECTION
40 – 43
Kristina Dunn's work of
art and style.

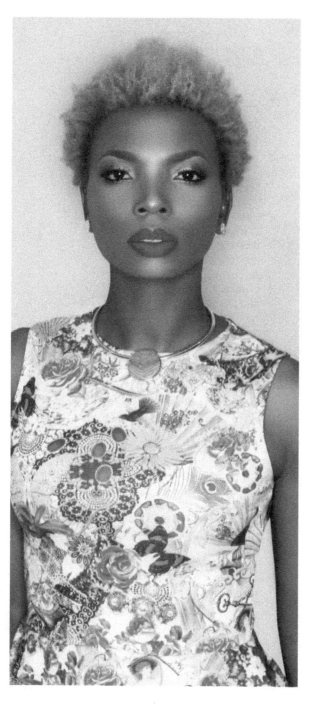

HAIR IDEAS
44 – 53
Looks you can wear
now!

STYLE NOTES
54 – 55
Quick and easy tips by
cosmetologist, Gabrielle
Roccuzzo.

PROTECTIVE STYLING
56 – 57
Ways to protect your
hair while sporting a
new look.

EARTH DAY
58 – 65
What is Earth Day? Plus
a photoshoot using
AVEDA's eco-friendly
products.

BRAID COLLECTION
66 – 69
Fun and creative braid
collection by Joël.

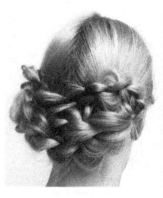

DIGITAL INFLUENCERS

Social Media got its big start in the late 90s early 2000's. Most social media sites were created so that users could talk to friends and family no matter where in the world they are located. YouTube and Facebook changed social media forever! The users are connecting through the sites which give the users a chance to know about each other cultures, fashion, music, and beauty tips that are used around the world. The bloggers/vloggers take their time getting to know a product then share their reviews to their viewers which leads to the viewer's feedback. That's really how consumers get to know what we love and hate about their products.

Digital Influencers are information omnivores who have spent time and effort building a loyal social media or web base. They have the ability to change opinions and behaviors. They are very active with social media, enhancing their position as opinion leaders.

We turned to several Digital Influencers to get the inside scoop on their style, their favorites, and more.

By: Ariel Johnson

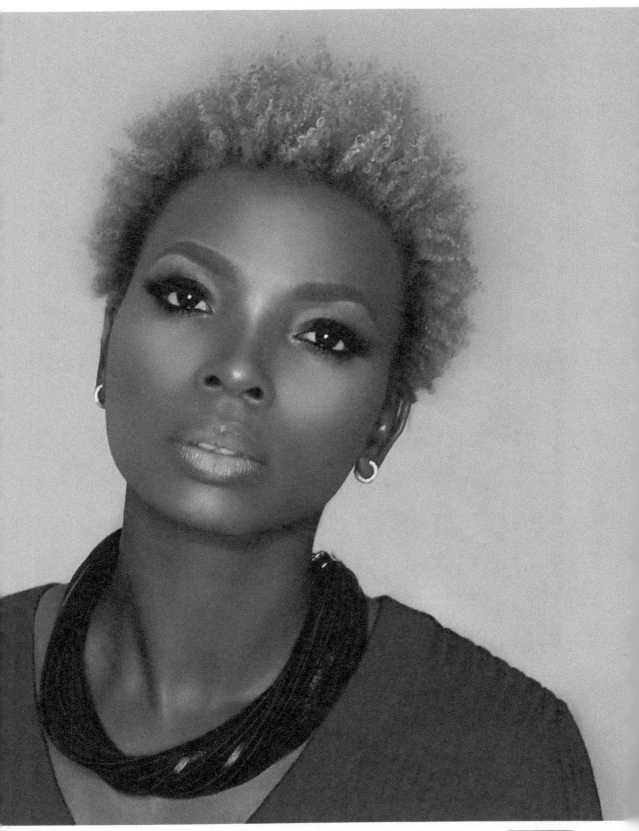

TYLA

This is my go-to wash n go style using Cantu leave in conditioner and curling creme. This is my go to style because it's easy and Cantu always helps my curls look their best. I split my hair in two and apply a generous amount of both products to both sections. After I apply the product and distribute evenly I diffuse my hair for 20 minutes until completely dry. After my hair is completely dry I pick my hair with a hair pick for extreme volume!

MY FAVORITE HAIR PRODUCTS
are Cantu's whole line of products. Including their leave in conditioner twist and lock gel and their curling creme. I also love Shea Moisture's black castor oil line for treatments and for retaining moisture and growth.

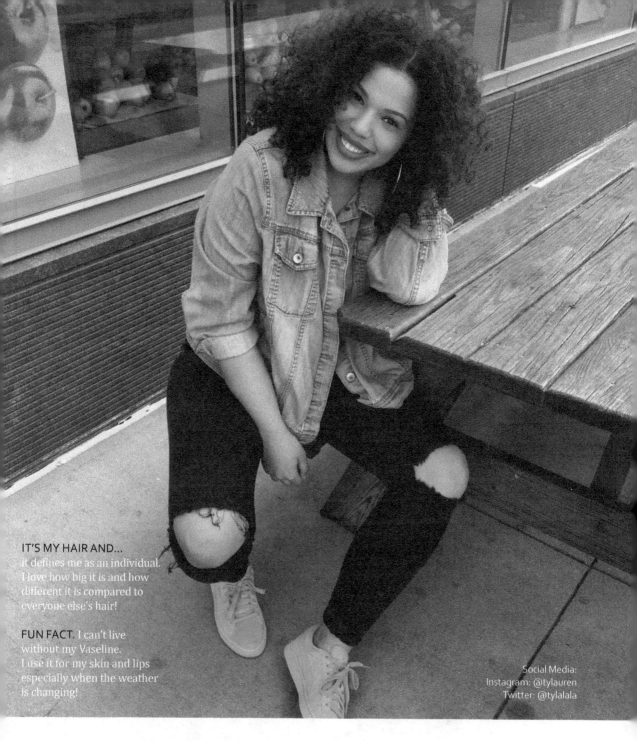

IT'S MY HAIR AND...
it defines me as an individual.
I love how big it is and how
different it is compared to
everyone else's hair!

FUN FACT. I can't live
without my Vaseline.
I use it for my skin and lips
especially when the weather
is changing!

Social Media:
Instagram: @tylauren
Twitter: @tylalala

I would describe my style as simple and comfortable. I'm always running around NYC for hours upon hours in a day so sneakers are my go to shoe. It thrifted both my jean jacket and black denim from Savers, thrift store in Rhode Island. My outfit in total costs me under $100 and I am always looking for deals and bargains because I hate spending a lot of money on clothes.

MY GO TO MAKEUP PRODUCTS *are MAC matte lipstick in the Taupe shade. I also love Maybelline's BB cream and Loreal's Infallible Foundation.*

MY FAVORITE HAIR TOOLS *include Deva Curls deva dryer and hair picks because I can't leave my house without it!*

IT'S MY HAIR AND...
it says that I am fearless.
It says that I am confident
in my own skin and refuse
to conform to anyone's
standard of beauty but
my own. It says that I am
fabulous and confident!

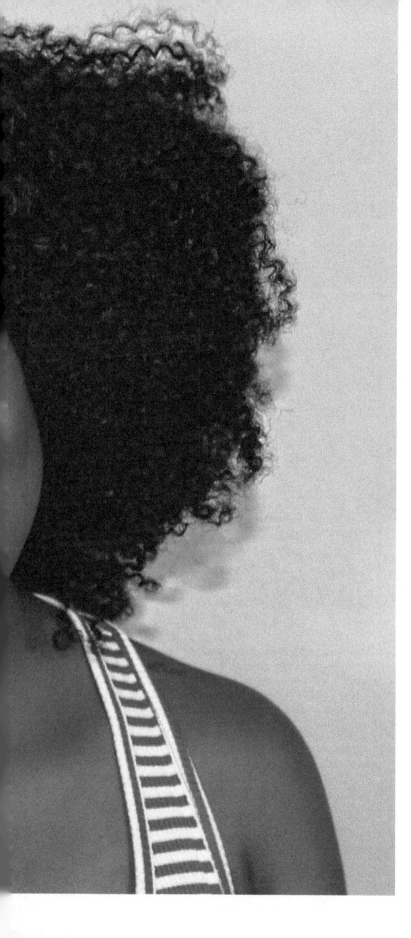

TROPHIE

I achieved this style with Her Given Hair natural hair extensions. To define my curls I used Creme of Nature Strength and Shine Leave-In Conditioner along with Shea Moisture JBCO Strengthen, Grow, and Restore Leave- In Conditioner. I used a Denman brush to make my curls pop and let my hair air dry. I then took down my flat twist and blended my natural hair with the extensions.

Youtube: trophdoph
Instagram: trophdoph
Snapchat: trophdoph
Twitter: trophdoph

BEAUTY FAVES.
Here are a couple of my favorite hair products: Shea Moisture JBCO Strengthen, Grow, and Restore Leave-In Conditioner, Beautiful Textures Rapid Repair Deep Conditioner, and the Giovanni Direct Leave-In Weightless Moisture Conditioner.

MY FAVORITE SKIN CARE PRODUCTS *are CeraVe foaming facial cleanser, CeraVe facial moisturizing lotion (am) and Natural Brand Aloe Vera Gel.*

MY FAVORITE MAKEUP PRODUCTS
are MakeupForever Ultra HD foundation, Mac Mineralized Skin Finish and Mac Blush in Raizin.

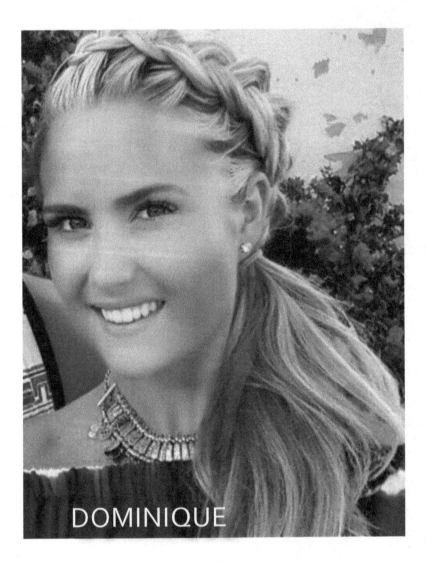

DOMINIQUE

DUTCH PONYTAIL. Dutch braids are such a summer hairstyle and I feel like they can really dress up an outfit too. They are basically an inside out French plait and are super quick and easy to do once you get the hang of them. I like to do them quite tight and then pull the braid out to make it appear nice and thick.

I like to accessorize using hair rings through the braid and love the Fudge urban scented hairsprays.

MY FAVORITE PRODUCTS
is the Unique One all in one hair treatment. It keeps my hair in tip-top shape and is amazing for detangling knotty hair like mine.

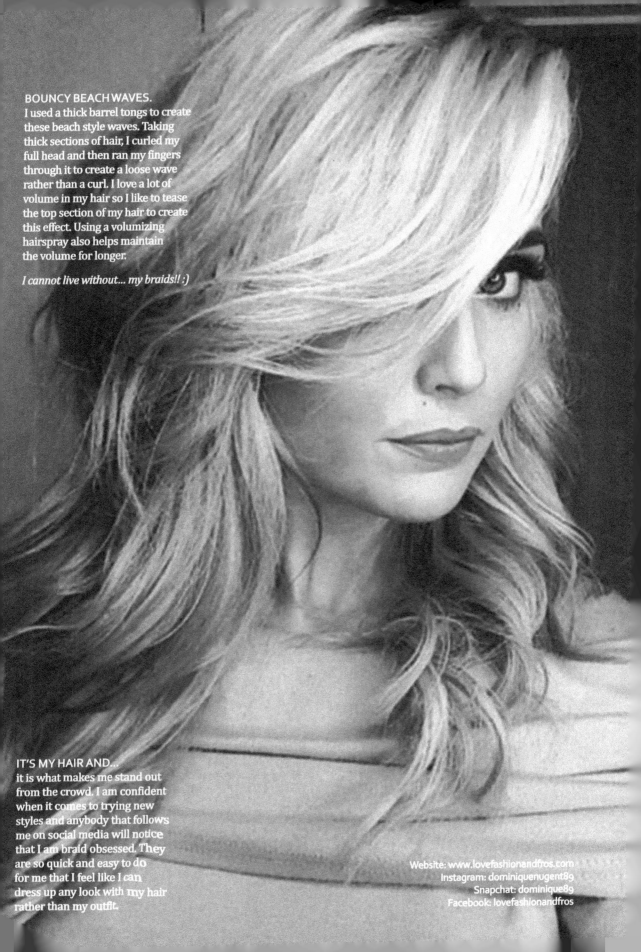

BOUNCY BEACH WAVES.
I used a thick barrel tongs to create these beach style waves. Taking thick sections of hair, I curled my full head and then ran my fingers through it to create a loose wave rather than a curl. I love a lot of volume in my hair so I like to tease the top section of my hair to create this effect. Using a volumizing hairspray also helps maintain the volume for longer.

I cannot live without... my braids!! :)

IT'S MY HAIR AND...
it is what makes me stand out from the crowd. I am confident when it comes to trying new styles and anybody that follows me on social media will notice that I am braid obsessed. They are so quick and easy to do for me that I feel like I can dress up any look with my hair rather than my outfit.

Website: www.lovefashionandfros.com
Instagram: dominiquenugent89
Snapchat: dominique89
Facebook: lovefashionandfros

SUSAN

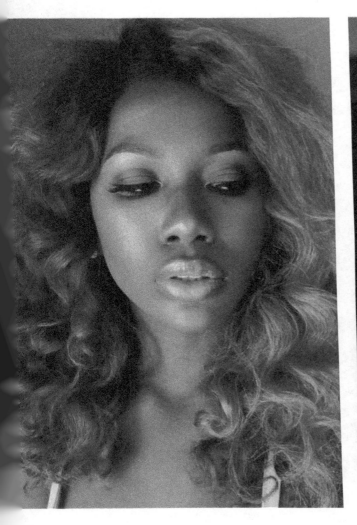 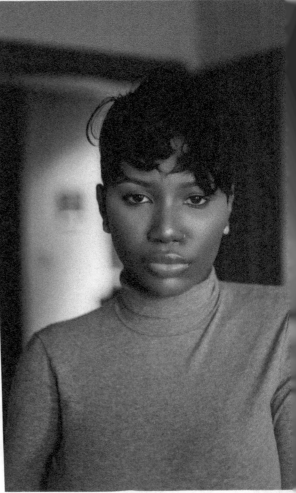

(left)

I call the first image fire and Ice. I chose this hairstyle because it was fiery and edgy. When I had this hairstyle I felt unstoppable and loved how it complimented my skin tone. This look was one of my favorite hairstyles.

(right)

I call the first image fire and Ice. I chose this hairstyle because it was fiery and edgy. When I had this hairstyle I felt unstoppable and loved how it complimented my skin tone. This look was one of my favorite hairstyles.

Instagram: @queen_suzie

IT'S MY HAIR AND...
it says that I am strong, brave and courageous. I love wearing my hair short and enjoy the flexibility of it. Because I wear my hair short, I often get a number of questions. I believe knowledge is the key to success so anytime I can take the opportunity to educate someone on natural hair I do just that. I believe that is what my hair says about me.

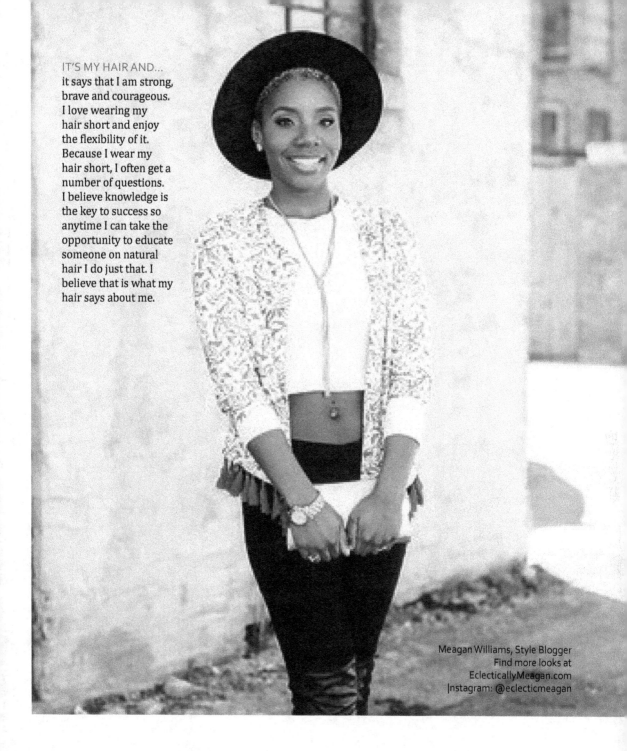

Meagan Williams, Style Blogger
Find more looks at
EclecticallyMeagan.com
Instagram: @eclecticmeagan

I love crop tops, so I knew I had to pair the top with this eclectic blazer. The tassels on the end make a bold statement. After adding the gold accessories, black velvet fedora and these black jeans with faux leather patches on the knees, I'm ready for a day out with my girls!

A FEW OF MY FAVORITE BEAUTY PRODUCTS *are Shea moisture Coconut & Hibiscus Brightening Body Lotion, Burt's Bees beeswax lip balm, Eden BodyWorks All Natural Cleansing Co-Wash, Stila Stay All Day Liquid Lipstick in the color "Beso".*

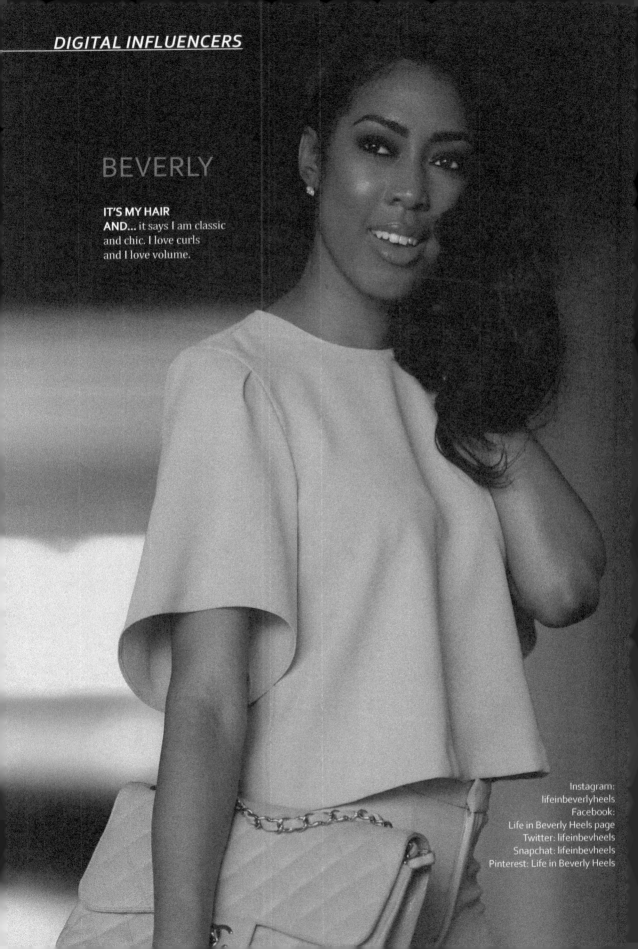

BEVERLY

IT'S MY HAIR AND... it says I am classic and chic. I love curls and I love volume.

Instagram: lifeinbeverlyheels
Facebook: Life in Beverly Heels page
Twitter: lifeinbevheels
Snapchat: lifeinbevheels
Pinterest: Life in Beverly Heels

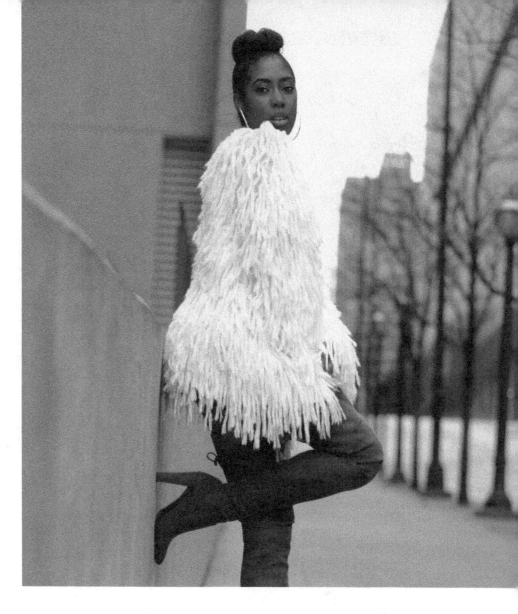

LOOK 1, page 14
This is a simple blow out look, my secret to having volume with my curls is that I don't fully press out my hair I curl my hair after its blow dried. (However this requires a really good blow dryer that does leave the hair straight but not pressed.)

LOOK 2, above
This look is a high bun. My secret is I spiral curl my entire head then put my hair in a bun. It's easier to work with and easier to pin.

SOME OF MY FAVE PRODUCTS
are MAC and Bobbi Brown.
I like to mix the foundations
together to get the perfect blend
for my complexion.

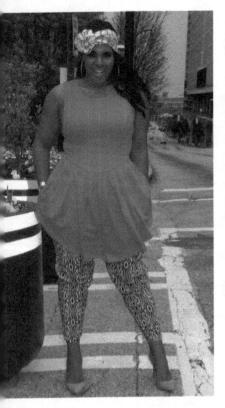 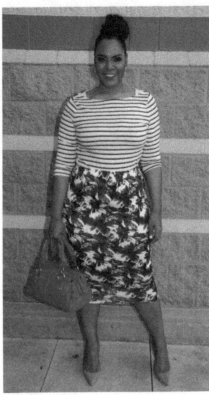 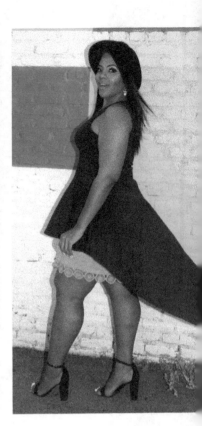

CRYSTAL

IT'S MY HAIR AND... it says that I am a carefree or a go with the flow type of girl! One day I want to wear my hair straight. Another day I will wear my natural curls. And the next day I like my hair in a messy bun! I do not take my hair too seriously.

BEACH WAVES: I love the look of effortless beauty. My go to style that I think can be casual or glam'd up are beach waves. I accomplish my beach wave hair style by using a curler wand. My hair generally does not keep curls so after I curl my hair I pin curl my curls to lock in the curls. Once I am ready to style, I take out my pin curls and run my fingers through my hair and let the curls fall naturally.

MESSY BUN: My everyday look is a messy bun. I put my hair in a loose ponytail and wrap my hair and pin it. Super easy.

FAVORITE PRODUCTS. *I use all Wen Hair products. I have tried countless hair brands, but Wen has completely transformed my hair from my hair growth, to the texture, defines my curls, and shine. I haven't found a skin care that I love. I am still on the search!*

MY FAVORITE HAIR STYLING TOOLS *is the flat iron and curler wand.*

HAIR ACCESSORIES. *I am obsessed with head scarves and wraps. I love to use my scarves as a fashion statement by mixing prints with my outfit. I love flower crowns. Finally, my go to is a hair bun donut, for quick and easy buns.*

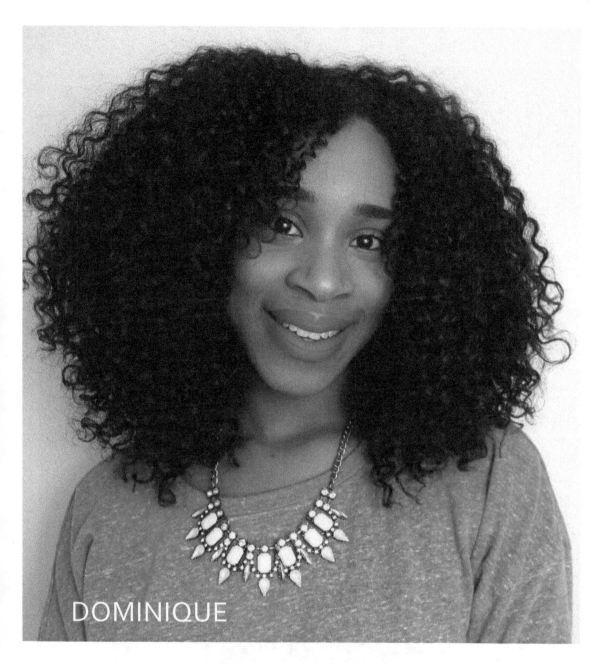

DOMINIQUE

The Wash and Go is probably my favorite natural hairstyle! It's a great feeling to finally figure out what products work for my hair but most of all, rocking a wash and go means I have accepted my hair in its natural curl pattern. This means accepting the great curl definition and frizziness. Both can be really frustrating at times. It's all beautiful!

SOME OF MY FAVORITE HAIR PRODUCTS *are Olive Oil Eco Styler Gel and Lotta Body Edge Control!*

FUN FACT: *I cannot live without my pick!*

BE SURE TO FIND ME ON SOCIAL MEDIA!
Instagram: @dommiekamelah | Snap Chat: xo_dommie | YouTube: Dommie Kamelah

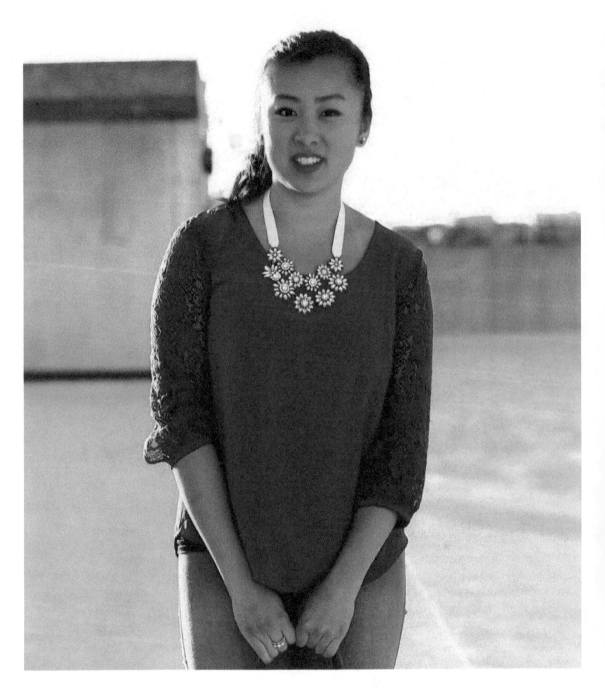

EMILY

LOOK 1 (above)
I've always loved statement necklaces and the way they can spice up any outfit! If you're looking to save a few dollars I recommend buying a white one from Baublebar because it'll last a long time and will match everything!

A FEW OF MY FAVORITE THINGS
HAIR: *Batiste dry shampoo, Conair Infiniti Curling Wand.* MAKEUP: *Smashbox Limitless Liquid Eyeliner, Naked2 palette.* SKINCARE: *Sephora Green Tea Eye Mask.*

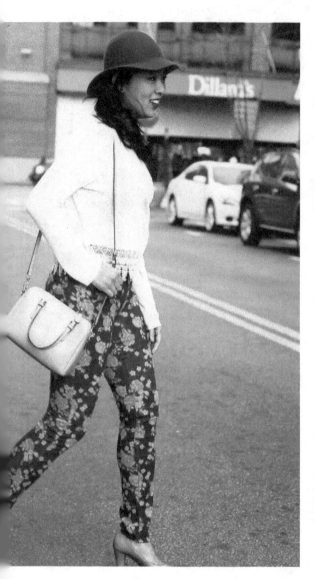
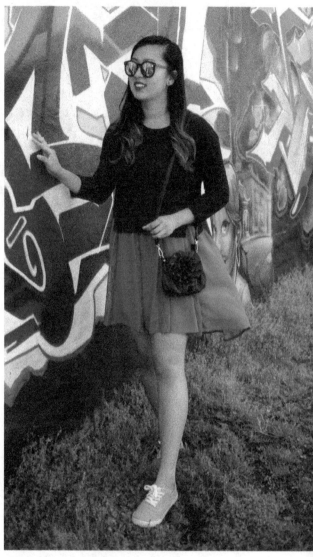

LOOK 2 (left)
Floral pants are the fastest way to look like you've given your outfit
a lot of thought when you haven't! I loved pairing these pants with
a floppy hat and nude heels!

LOOK 3 (right)
My favorite looks lately are effortless, street style looks. My gray sneakers
are an essential for making any outfit super casual.

CONNECT WITH ME:
Twitter/Facebook/Instagram: @emsies_Emily | www.emsies.com

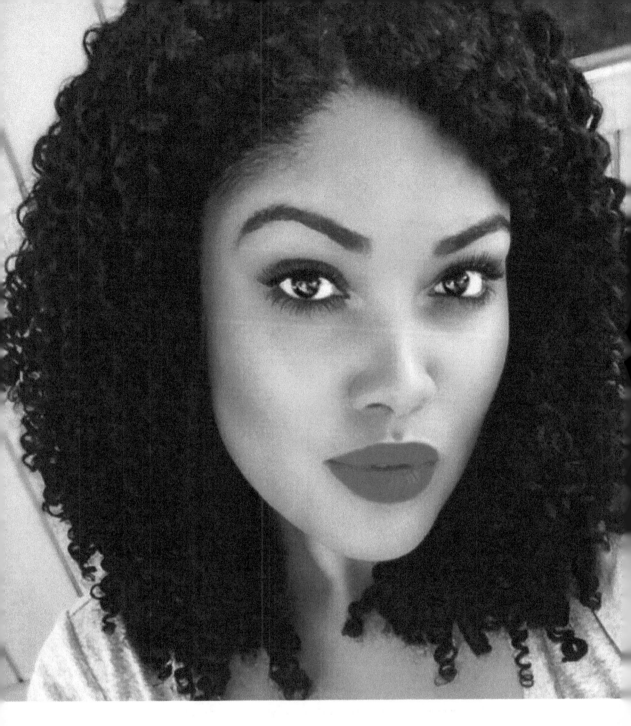

CANDACE

My signature style is the "Wash and Go" but recently I've discovered how to successfully pull off the "Braid and Curl". To achieve this style, I start on freshly washed hair. I use any cream based twist or braid cream that I have available and apply a small amount to each section of hair. I create about 15-18 braids, leave about an inch of hair unbraided at the ends and apply a small perm rod. I let the style dry and set overnight. The next day, I remove the perm rods, unravel the braids and fluff with my hair pick. That's it! The "Braid and Curl" is a new favorite!

by Candice Crocker

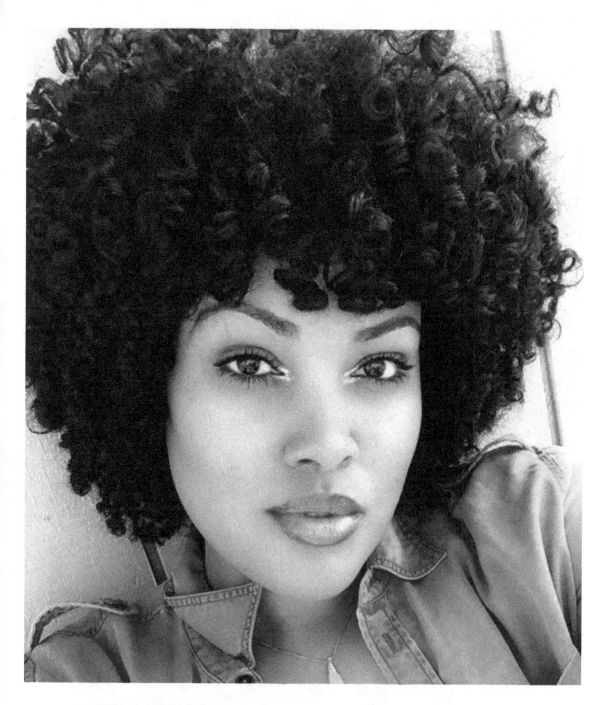

I CANNOT LIVE WITHOUT MY...

Dramatically Different Moisturizing Lotion+ from Clinique. My mother began purchasing it for me when I was in high school and it's the best face lotion I've ever tried. Absolute staple!

SOCIAL MEDIA:
Instagram: @candicoatedcurls | YouTube: youtube.com/candicearielle

FAVORITE HAIR PRODUCTS:

Kinky Curly Knot Today, Olive Oil Ecostyler Gel
Aussie 3 Minute Miracle Moist Deep Conditioner

FAVORITE MAKEUP PRODUCTS:

Pro Longwear Nourishing Waterproof
Foundation by MAC
Becca Cosmetics Shimmering Skin Perfector
in Champagne Pop
Benefit Cosmetics They're Real Mascara

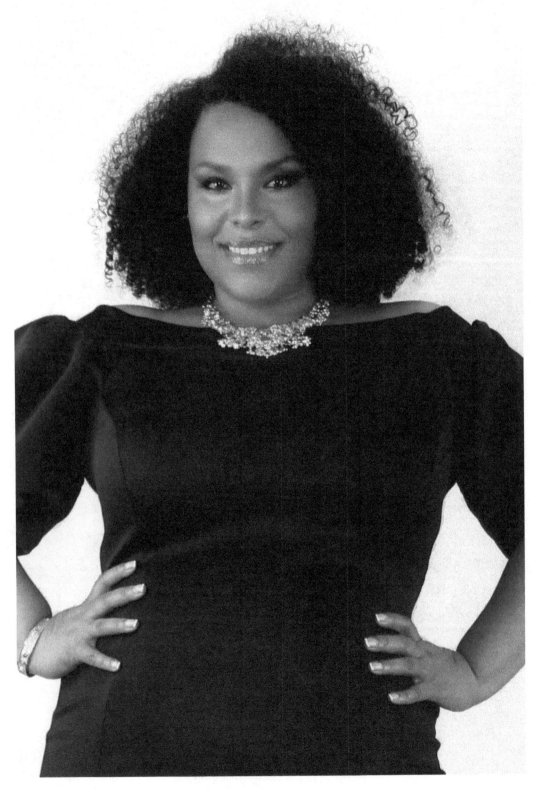

Makeup: Robert Guy, on Instagram @therguy
Photographer: LASEWOD Photography
(left & right)

FRO'S AND WASH N' GO'S

Over the decades, black communities have been handed everything to control what others see as nappy. From hot combs to relaxer creams our tresses has witness it all. But, in the late 1950s and early 1960s, a shift took place that would change the way we see ourselves forever, the Afro. The afro is freshly washed hair combed out from the roots to the ends and formed in a circular shape. The black community first started the natural transition during the Civil Right movement. The afro signified self-worth, confidence, and enlightened the world to know that we see ourselves for who we are truly.

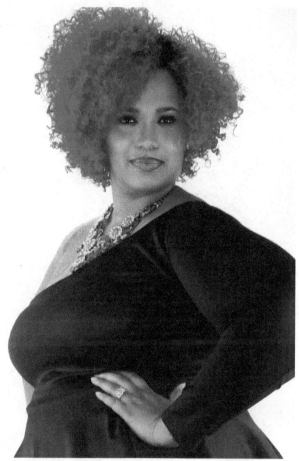

During the time of transitioning from straight to natural the styles became pretty creative. While most women were wearing the fro, others were rocking the wash and go. This style consists of a fresh shampoo and condition to the hair and then go as you please! Others were transitioning by wearing braids and beads. Either rocking them individually or braided to the scalp, this style is always a plus. Then there are the women who loves to twist their hair at night and unravel in the a.m. for a stylish twist out that leaves the tress with flawless curls. All the styles stated above are not only stylish but also protects the hair and helps produce growth.

As we are still transitioning from straight to natural our minds are also growing through the same phase. Evolving to love our hair naturally and protectively all the while being creative and stylish.

By: Ariel Johnson

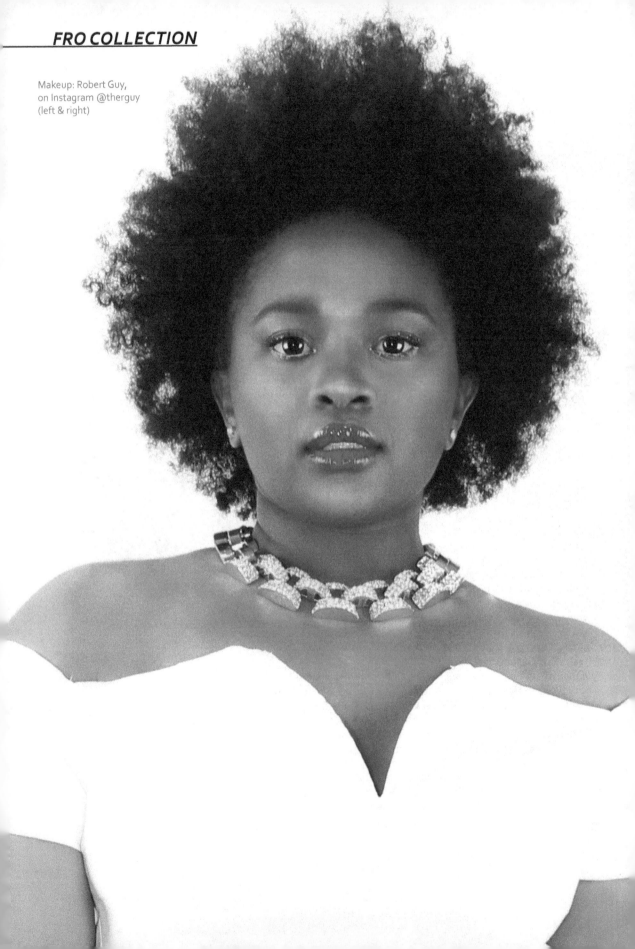

Makeup: Robert Guy,
on Instagram @therguy
(left & right)

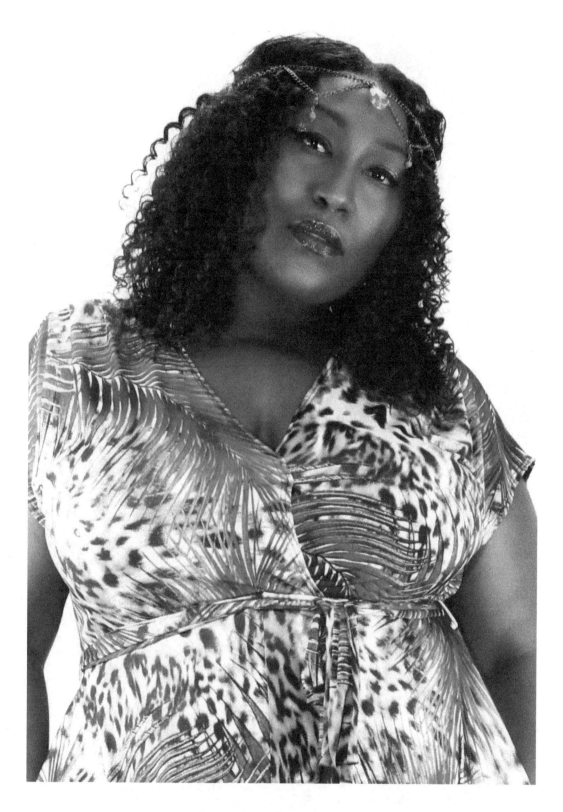

Photographer: LASEWOD Photography
(left & right)

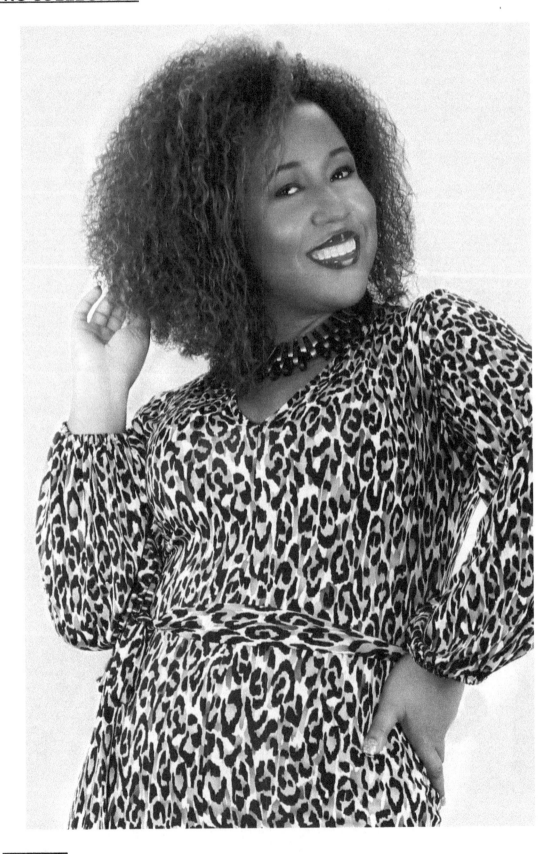

Makeup: Robert Guy,
on Instagram @therguy (left)
Photographer:
LASEWOD Photography
(left & right)

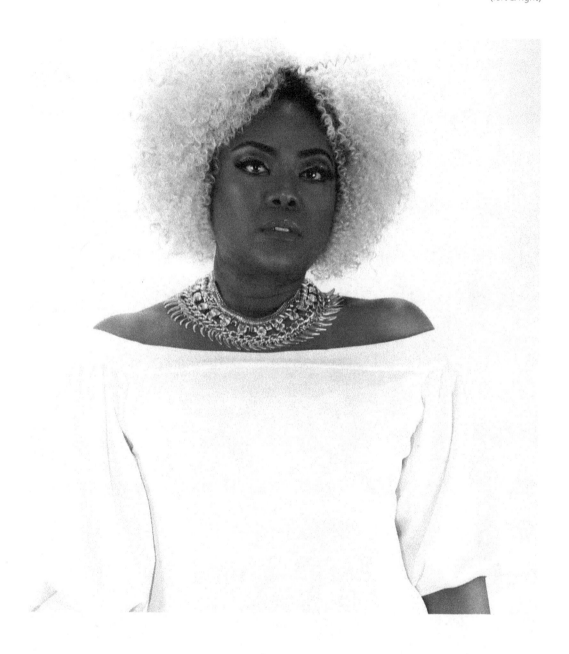

Jalese Ayana, A.K.A LEESY

FUN FACTS - I Got on an airplane for the first time when I was 19. I consider myself
to be an all around creative, using photography, music, film, fine art, and fashion as mediums.
I would've NEVER thought I would be wearing an Afro if somebody asked me 3 years ago.

Social Media: @Jalese.Ayana (personal Instagram) or @leesythooo (Photography instagram)
Website: www.Leesytho.com

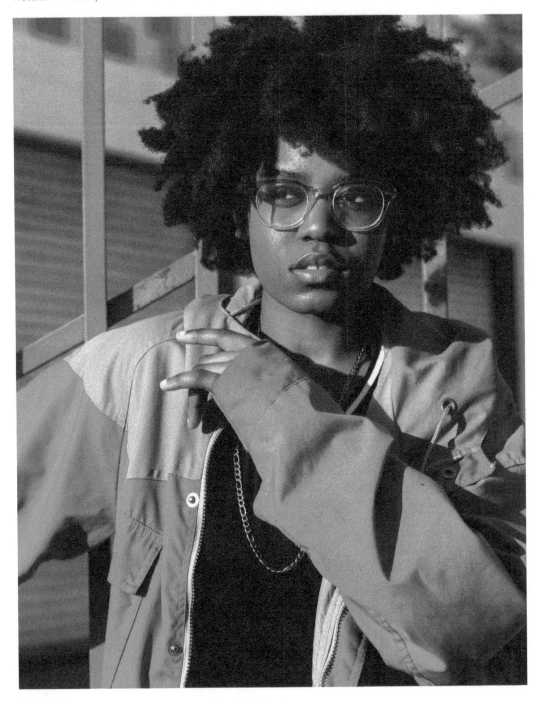

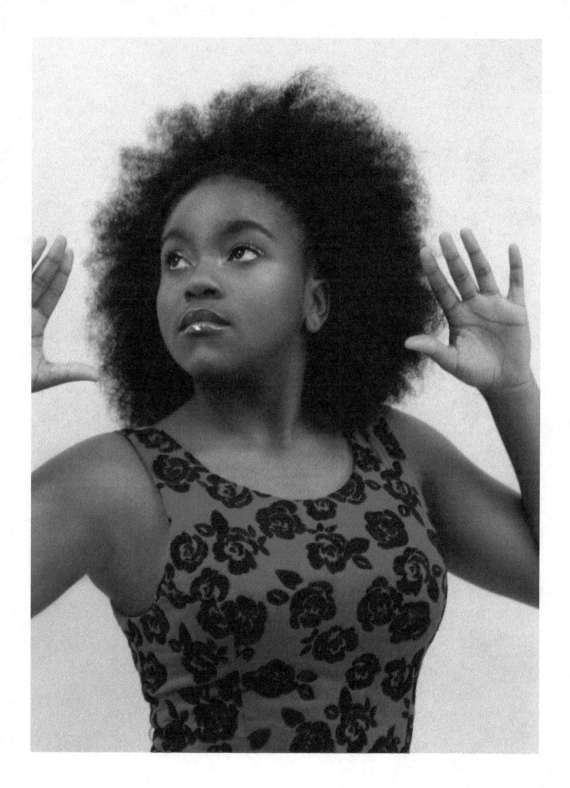

Makeup: Robert Guy, on Instagram @therguy
Photographer: LASEWOD Photography

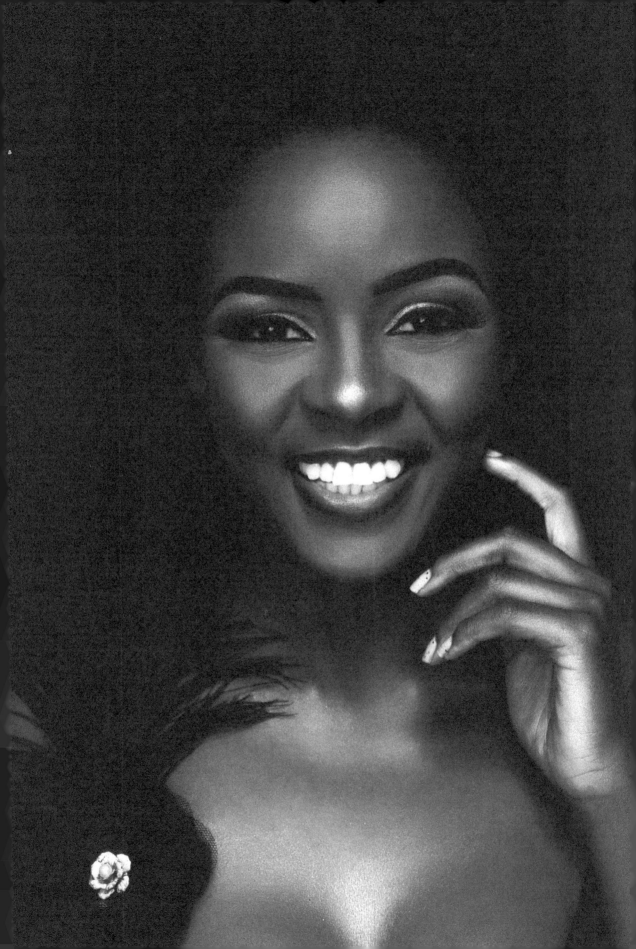

WHO IS SHEILA NDINDA?

I am fun-loving, creative and energetic naturalista, born and raised up in Nairobi Kenya. I partly run a Natural hair and Beauty blog by the name African Tresses and Treats and also have a YouTube Channel. I spend the rest of my days at my full time job, the Capital Club East Africa, a private business club where I work as a Membership Manager.

WHO WOULD BE YOUR ULTIMATE SOCIAL MEDIA INFLUENCER TO MEET?

Oh my, this a hard one. I would definitely say Jackie Aina. She is a You tuber and a makeup guru. I absolutely love the way she incorporates humor into all her videos. Her channel is filled with tons of makeup tutorials and product reviews which always helps me to keep track of the new makeup trends in every season. She is also my natural hair sister.

Jackie is a gorgeous dark skinned beauty, who inspires me a lot because she is very successful, ever smiling (even when people criticize her) and role model for all the young women out there.

She is a woman who loves her beautiful dark skin and teaches me to embrace and love the skin that I am in.

WHY DID YOU START A BLOG?

I was a baldie growing up as it was mandatory for all the students to be bald in the school I attended. I remember being super depressed. I thought I was very ugly because I did not have any strands of hair. Years later in high school, I was finally able to wear my hair out but it was convenient for me to relax it. My hair slowly weakened and started breaking. I then started researching on how I could rock my hair in its natural hair state and a few weeks later, I did the big chop.

I started my blog as my natural hair journal to document my personal journey into learning how to take care of my hair and how to style it. I wanted to connect with other naturalistas and be a source of inspiration to women thinking of going natural by offering support, sharing tips and experiences throughout my journey.

With the lack of many International Natural Hair products brands in Kenya, I saw my blog as a platform for me to share with other naturals on locally available products and how to incorporate them into their natural hair regimen. I developed the urge to start helping my viewers understand their natural hair and provide them with information and resources to naturally achieve healthy natural hair. I also saw it as a platform to show them "how tos" how to do this, how to do that.

My blog has given me the opportunity to showcase my likes and dislikes and also my favorite beauty products.

WHAT IS YOUR HIDDEN TALENT?

I am an amazing cook! Unlike most Kenyan families, we did not have a househelp growing up and so I was usually the one assigned kitchen duties. I learnt to make a number of delicacies and I have to admit now it's more fun than it was back then.

I find myself experimenting a lot, good thing it always leads up to yet another tasty meal.

MOST PLAYED SONG ON YOUR ITUNES/MP3/PHONE, ETC.?

I can listen to What Do You Want Me To Do by Rihanna over and over again.

FIVE THINGS YOU ALWAYS KEEP IN YOUR BEAUTY BAG?

Maybelline Mascara - I love Mascaras because they instantly brighten up my eyes. Most of the time, it's the only make up I wear, and it really does make a difference.

Mac Studio fix Concealer –They come in handy when I want to hide any blemishes and dark circles, eye bugs that appear on my skin. I find that this particular concealer gives me the perfect coverage.

Mac Studio Fix powder plus foundation – This is ideal for me because it gives my skin a flawless matte finish.

EOS Lip Blam to keep my lips soft, smooth and moisturized. Nobody wants to walk around with chapped or cracked lips. They are not attractive at all and are always painful if not taken care of.

Revlon Super Lustrous Lipstick in Mink which is a neutral everyday lipstick. The nude color compliments my skin tone. I love its natural and subtle look.

Sleek Face Foam Kit in medium - I use the highlighter just above my cheekbones and on the bridge of my nose. It adds such a beautiful glow for everyday makeup.

BOYFRIEND?

Yes I do have a boyfriend. He is everything I ever wished for in a man.

WHAT QUALITIES DO YOU LOOK FOR IN A GUY?

A respectful and principled man. He should be intelligent, open minded and above all ambitious.

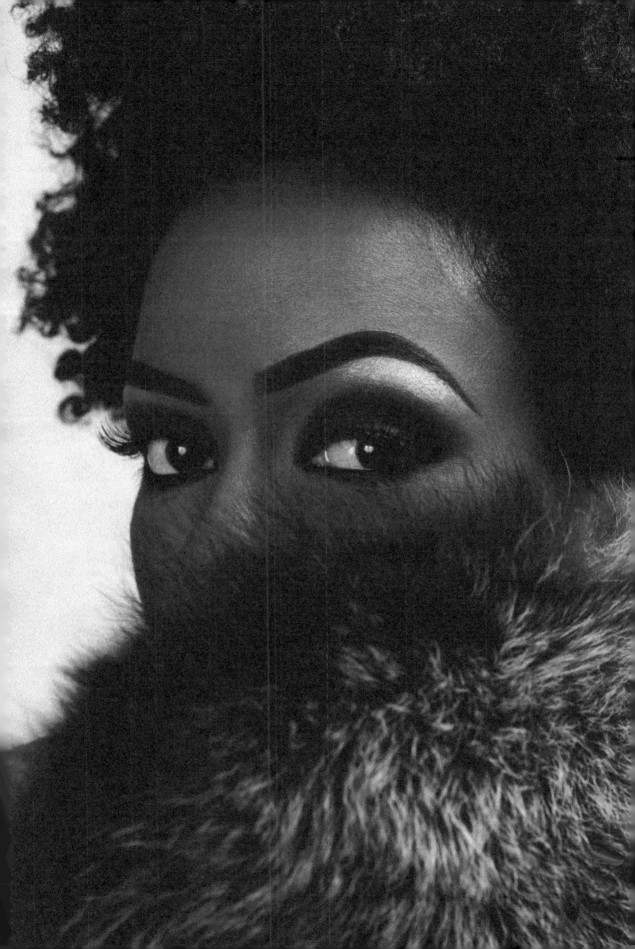

Sheila

STYLE ICON IN FASHION?
Kyrzayda Rodriguez of www.kyrzayda.com who is well known for her fierce haircut, fit physique and impeccable sense of style.

I adore her chic but fun style. Her outfit's coordination is very well put together. She combines unique pieces and tones them down with sleek lines of suede and knits.

SIGNATURE HAIR STYLE?
Twist outs. You can never go wrong with a twist out. I have also mastered the art of making my twists last a week long which relieves me from the stress of having to retwist every night.

FAVORITE PERFUME?
PacoRabanne in Lady Million. I would describe this fragrance as a perfect perfume for every day wear. It's feminine yet playful and I think it's a real acquisition in my perfume stash.

GO-TO HAIR STYLE?
My go-to hair style is Bantu knots because they are easy to do and I love how my strands are transformed to a curly fro with minimal effort.

FAVORITE HAIR PRODUCTS.
Shea by Asal Shampoo bar is my favorite shampoo hands down. It contains bentonite clay which is an excellent cleanser. It does not strip my hair too much of its natural moisture.

Ajani Handmade waridi butter – which I use a sealant or a cream to moisturize and style my hair. It has the perfect not too creamy consistency and makes my hair super moisturized.

Coconut Oil – I mix it with my deep conditioner for a moisture boost. I also use it to prepoo my hair before washing and also mix it with other natural oils for a hot oil treatment which promotes shiny hair.

Shea Moisture 10 in 1 renewal system superfruit complex Deep conditioner- It contains Biotin and Marula oil which helps promote healthy hair. It leaves my dry hair feeling so soft, vibrant and looking shiny.

Tropical Isle Jamaican Castor Oil– I use it do to Scalp massages. It's perfect for blood circulation that *helps to promote hair growth.*

Cantu Coconut Curling Cream - It smells like a dream!! It's really moisturizing, does not flake and defines the hell out of my curls hehe. It's perfect for my twist outs and braid outs.

#1 ON YOUR BUCKET LIST.
I am actually dreaming about Santorini, Greece.

WHO ARE SOME OF YOUR FAVORITE BLOGGERS?
Askproy
She is my absolute favorite and was my inspiration to getting my tapered cut. I love that she gets across to so many women just through her you tube channel and blog and that's one of the most important things about blogging. She loves to experiment with a variety of hairstyles including Perm rod sets, twist outs, braid outs and also plays around with hair colors. Her hairstyles are definitely an eye catcher.

Sola of Discovering Naturals
Her you tube channel provides information about natural hair care. It shows different product reviews, and "how-to" videos experimenting with different products. Her channel also showcases hair routines for her kids where she is always teaching them to embrace and love their natural hair.

Jenell Stewart aka blakizbeautyful
I have been watching her videos before I even decided to go natural. She does lots of product reviews and offers great styling tips which are a perfect guide to a healthy hair journey.

Jessica Pettway
Her channel has a variety of hairstyles. She shares with viewers how to DIY weaves and wigs and how to blend them with their natural hair. And she has such an adorable daughter whom she is always parading on YouTube. Love her!

Ambrosia Malbrough
I am obsessed with her natural beauty and humble personality. She has gorgeous hair and shares tips on how to maintain and style it on her YouTube channel and vlogs. She also designs jewelry, and documents her tips on living a minimal and chic lifestyle. Let's not forget her glowy skin that always gives me the Goosebumps.

FAVORITE FOOD
My favorite food is Fish. I can have it in any form or shape really and at any time of the day. Thank God for fish, lol.

COUNTRIES TRAVELED.
I have not been fortunate enough to travel around; I have only been to South Africa, Uganda, Tanzania and will be travelling to London in September.

THE INTERVIEW

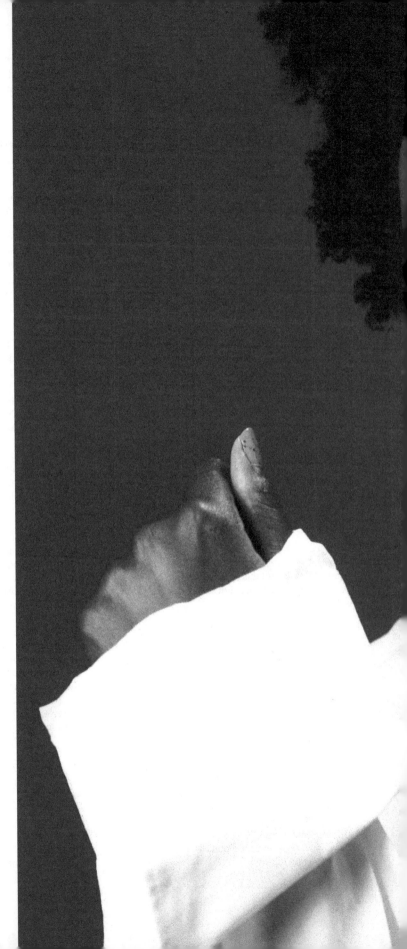

CREDITS PAGES 30 THROUGH 37
Photographer: Lyra Aoka
on Instagram @lyraoko
Website: www.lyraoko.com
Makeup Artist: Joy Balogun
on Instagram @sunshinebalogun
Website: www.sunshinebalogun.com

FIND ME
Blog - www.africantressesandtreats.com
You Tube - Sheila Ndinda
Instagram @sheilandinda
Facebook - African Tresses and Treats

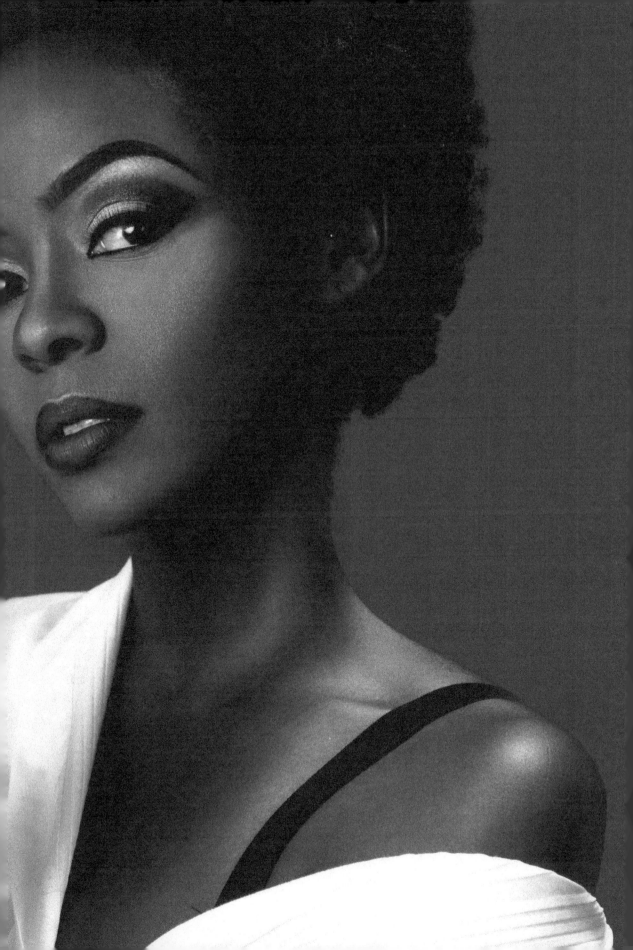

WHAT IS A MISCONCEPTION ABOUT KENYA?
One of the biggest misconceptions I have noticed is that Kenyans, all Kenyans, want to live abroad because they believe life is better off and there are better opportunities there.

Like any other society there are those who hold this belief, but many Kenyans would rather stay back home and work on building themselves and their families rather than go away to some other country full of strangers and start basically from nothing. With the growth of infrastructure and technology in Kenya, many people realize they can actually make it while right here. And besides, the internet has made the world smaller and east or west home is always best.

WHAT IS A REALLY BAD HABIT THAT YOU WANT TO BREAK?
Taking "no" for an answer without trying again.

HAVE YOU PICKED UP ANY STYLE TIPS FROM YOUR FAVORITE BLOGGERS?
Yes absolutely! *P Roy* made me fall in love with perm rod sets

Ambrosia Malbrough has taught me to take a minimalistic approach while stocking up my closet.

There is genius in Simplicity.

WHAT HAIR PRODUCT BRANDS ARE YOU LOYAL TO?
Shea Moisture, even though the products are costly and hard to get in Kenya, I always find a way of getting my hands on some. My hair loves their deep conditioning treatments.

HAVE YOU EXPERIENCED SOCIAL MEDIA BULLYING OR BODY SHAMING? HOW DID YOU HANDLE IT?
Honestly, I cannot say I have. I have been lucky to have a supportive fan base all through my journey. I believe I am Real as a person and everything I put out is 100% me. I am also from the school of thought that if you are comfortable in your own skin and with who you are as a person then you leave no room for bullies and characters who are into body shaming.

That said, I believe it is very bad and should be stopped by all means necessary. I am all about the positive vibes both on and off the internet.

WHAT IS THE MOST MEANINGFUL THING SOMEONE HAS EVER SAID TO YOU?
I get a lot of people telling me I inspire them when it comes to going natural and in their day to day lives in general. This makes me aware that the little things you do have an impact on someone somewhere no matter how small.

WHAT DOES YOUR HAIR SAY ABOUT YOU?
I am an extrovert and very playful person. I am open to new experiences and not afraid to go for what I want in life. I wasn't always like this and I believe wearing my hair the way I want gave me the confidence to explore myself more and accentuate the characteristics that define me today.

WHY DO YOU LOVE IT'S MY HAIR! MAGAZINE?
I love it because it advocates for women embracing their inner beauty and obviously because it is about my favorite subject; hair.

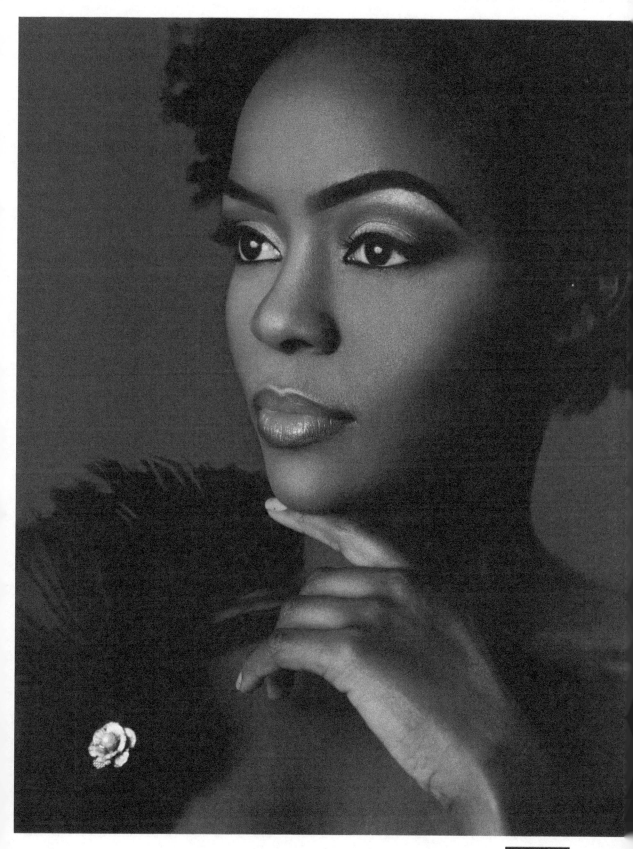

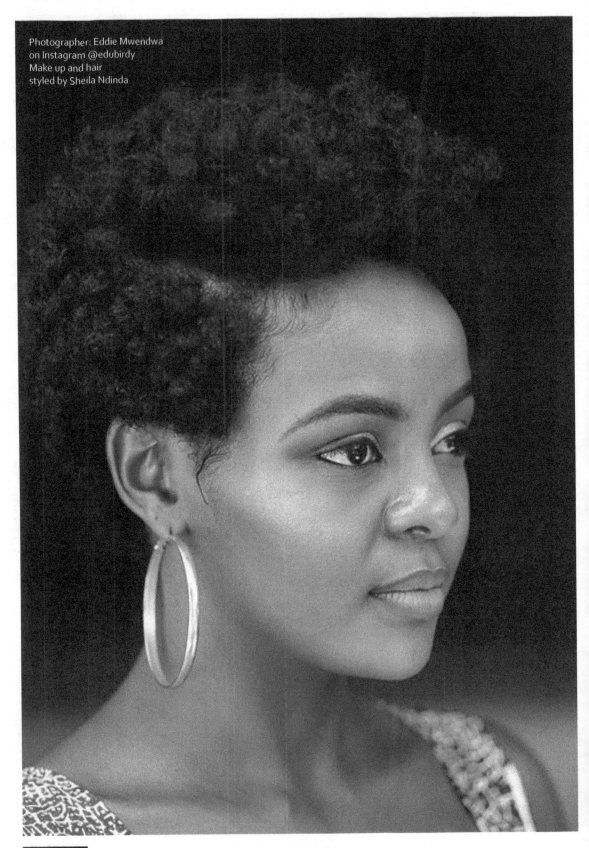

Photographer: Eddie Mwendwa
on Instagram @edubirdy
Make up and hair
styled by Sheila Ndinda

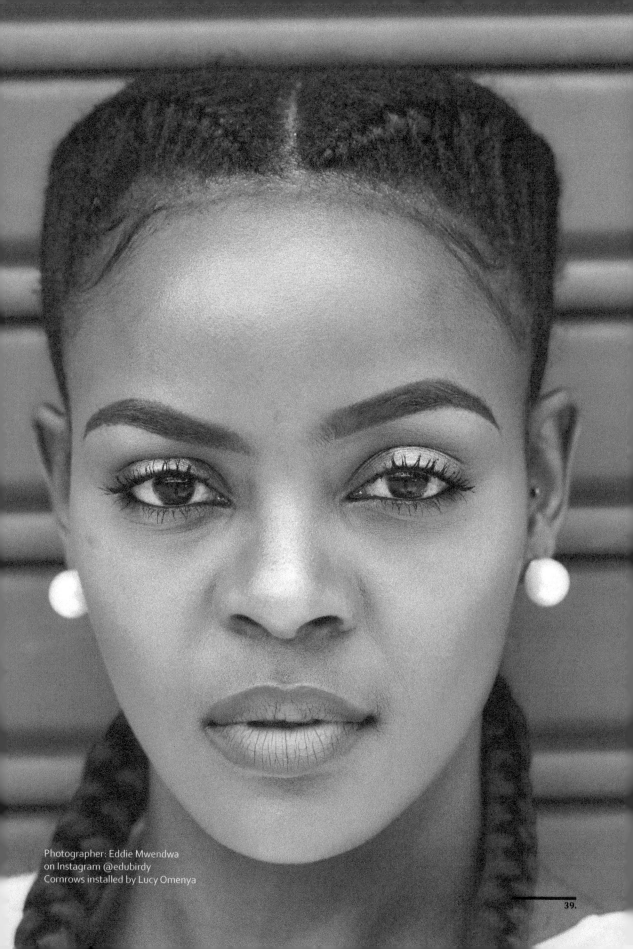

Photographer: Eddie Mwendwa
on Instagram @edubirdy
Cornrows installed by Lucy Omenya

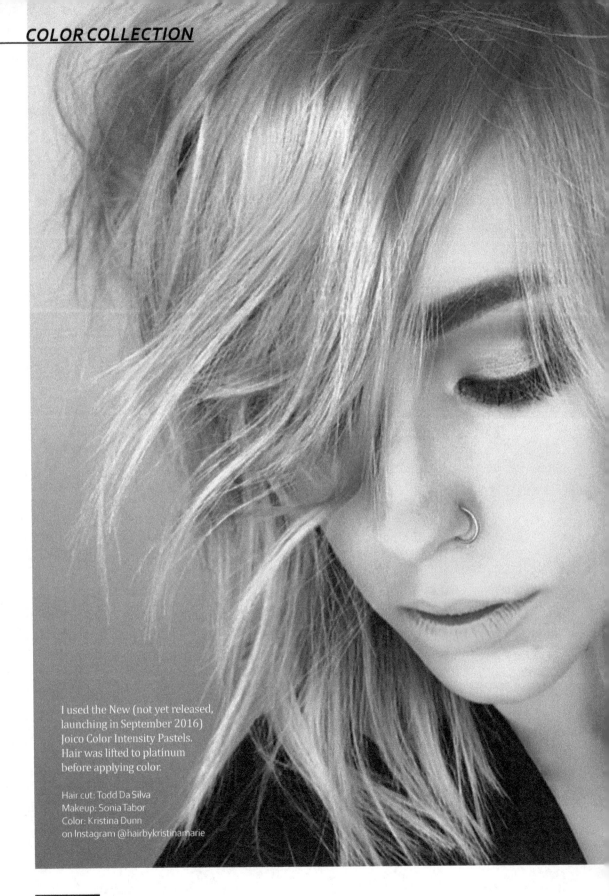

I used the New (not yet released, launching in September 2016) Joico Color Intensity Pastels. Hair was lifted to platinum before applying color.

Hair cut: Todd Da Silva
Makeup: Sonia Tabor
Color: Kristina Dunn
on Instagram @hairbykristinamarie

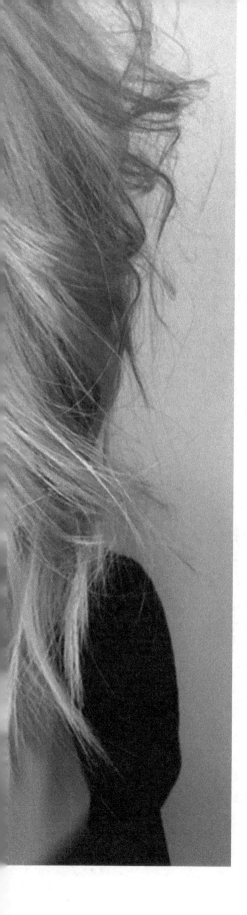

Here at IT'S MY HAIR MAGAZINE, *we love to involve ourselves with the best and Kristina Dunn is the best at what she does. Each hair masterpiece is bold, vibrant and rich in flavor. Dunn techniques will provide you with the wonderful vibes that all girls want to feel when leaving out the salon, especially that confident feeling.*

By Ariel Johnson

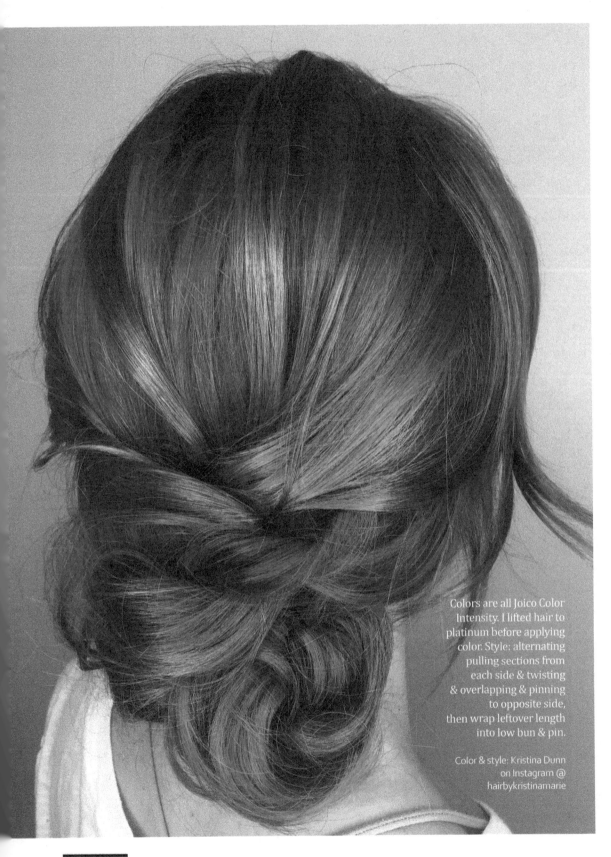

Colors are all Joico Color Intensity. I lifted hair to platinum before applying color. Style: alternating pulling sections from each side & twisting & overlapping & pinning to opposite side, then wrap leftover length into low bun & pin.

Color & style: Kristina Dunn on Instagram @ hairbykristinamarie

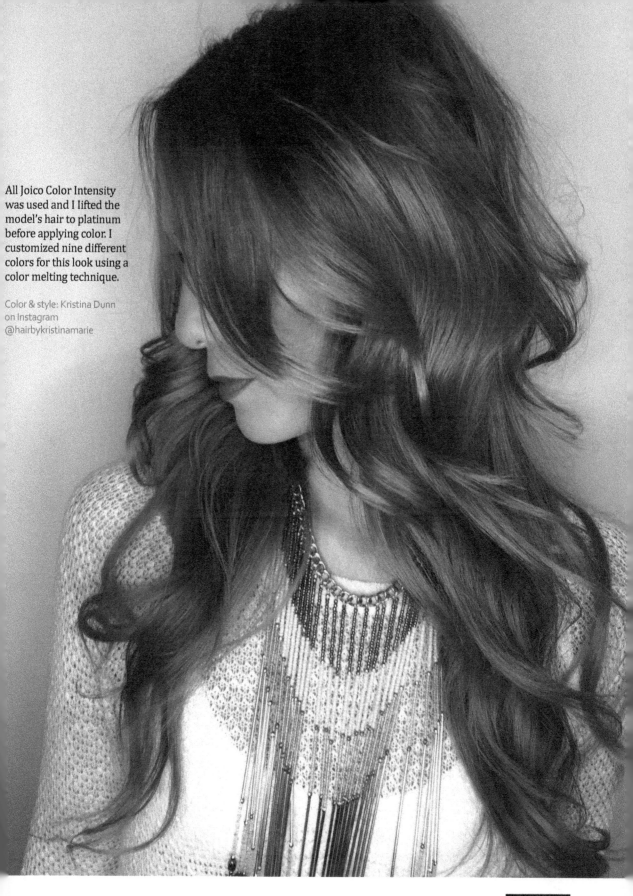

All Joico Color Intensity was used and I lifted the model's hair to platinum before applying color. I customized nine different colors for this look using a color melting technique.

Color & style: Kristina Dunn
on Instagram
@hairbykristinamarie

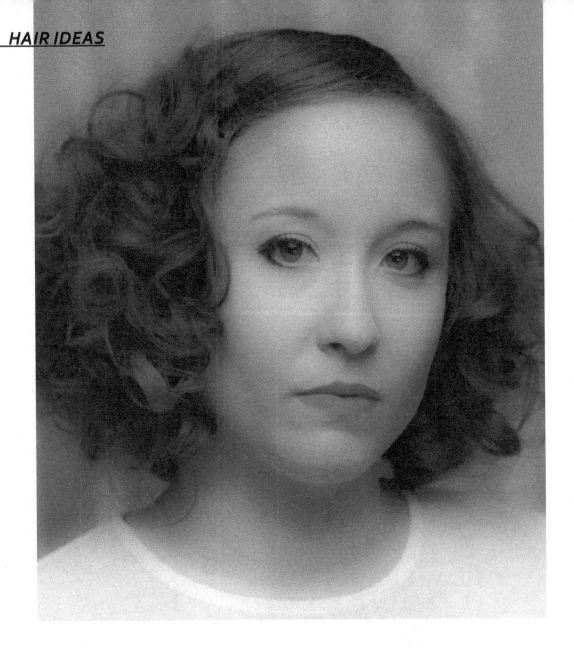

*Tight curls on long length hair
using flat irons on 450 degrees
and rolled on flexi-rods overnight.
Created custom color using 7RR by Croma
and 30% developer.*

Styled by Sherrie Cheriel's Hair Gallery,
on Instagram @sherriecheriel
Makeup by Maniele Banks,
on Instagram @pressplay87
Photography by CR142 Photos,
www.cr142photos.com

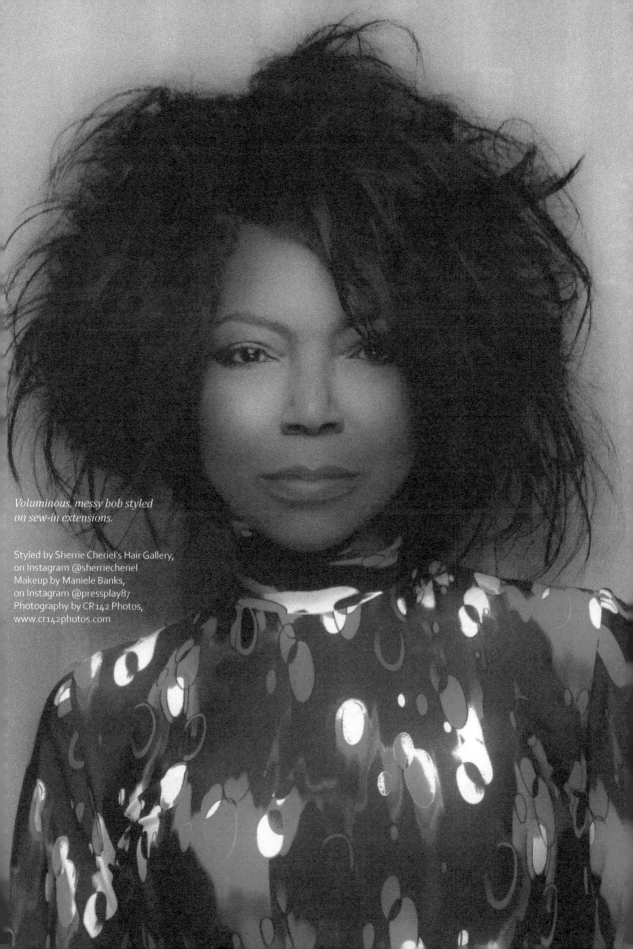

*Voluminous, messy bob styled
on sew-in extensions.*

Styled by Sherrie Cheriel's Hair Gallery,
on Instagram @sherriecheriel
Makeup by Maniele Banks,
on Instagram @pressplay87
Photography by CR142 Photos,
www.cr142photos.com

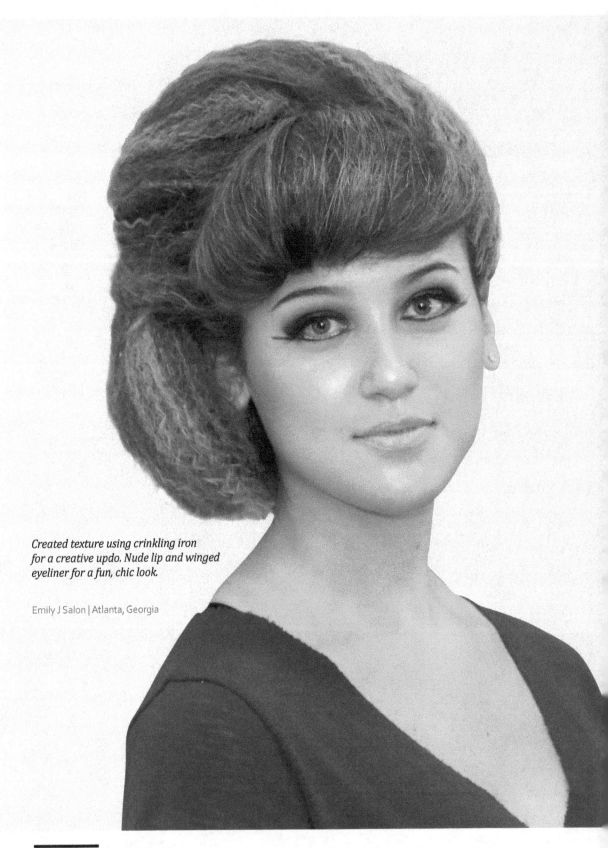

Created texture using crinkling iron for a creative updo. Nude lip and winged eyeliner for a fun, chic look.

Emily J Salon | Atlanta, Georgia

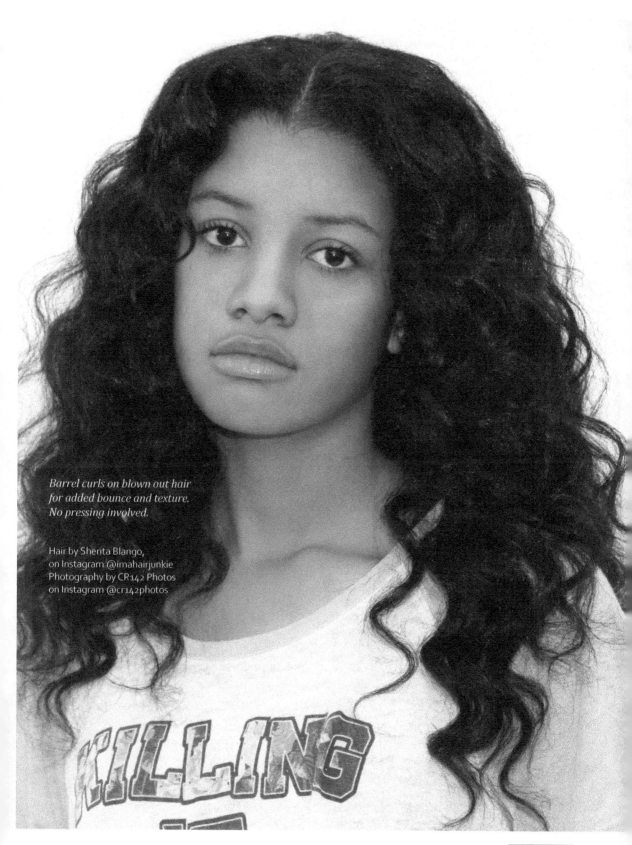

Barrel curls on blown out hair
for added bounce and texture.
No pressing involved.

Hair by Sherita Blango,
on Instagram @imahairjunkie
Photography by CR142 Photos
on Instagram @cr142photos

HAIR IDEAS

Hats are considered fashion accessories
that set you apart if worn correctly. Here the model
wears a stylish hat with a patterned dress.
It features a neutral color that flatters her skin and
the slightly dipped brim brings focus to her face.

Wardrobe Stylist: Sharon Edwards
Courtesy of LASEWOD Photography

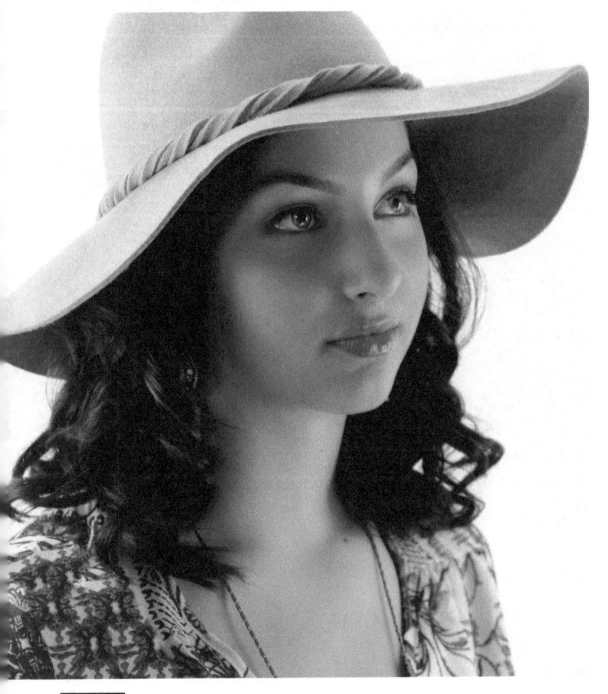

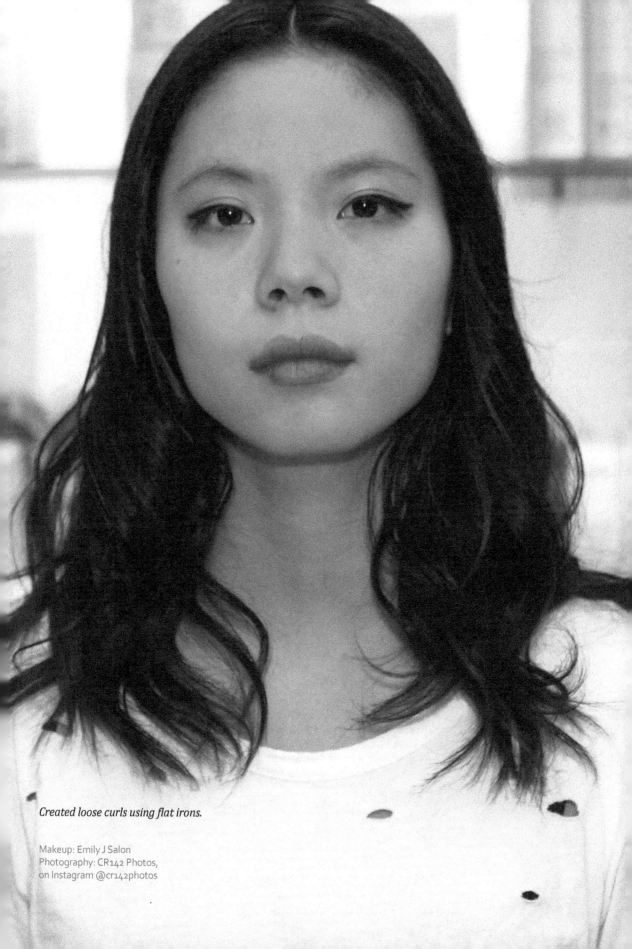

Created loose curls using flat irons.

Makeup: Emily J Salon
Photography: CR142 Photos,
on Instagram @cr142photos

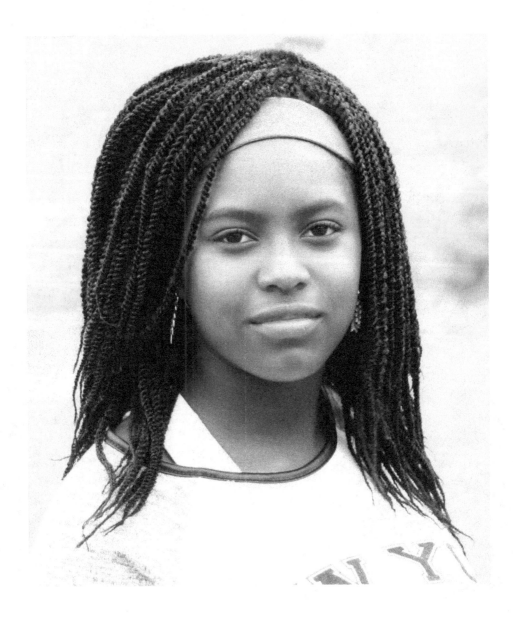

Crochet techniques have come a long ways from the
90's with the help of YouTube and Instagram. They
are really popular for providing styling options for
almost any look. So if you are looking for a hands off
approach, protective style or simply want a new do
then crochet braids is the way to go

Braids by Kristi Lathon Kudotorres@yahoo.com
on Instagram @mama.kudo
Photography: LASEWOD Photography,
on Instagram @lasewod_photography

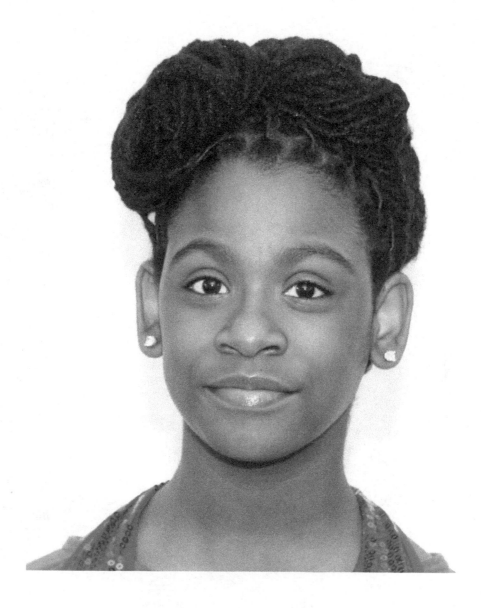

Loc'd hair is gathered strands of hair that has not been combed or brushed and left alone to mat together. The model in this photo has shoulder length locs styled into a gorgeous updo.

Styled by Sherita Blango,
on Instagram @imahairjunkie
Photography: CR 142 Photos,
www.cr142photos.com

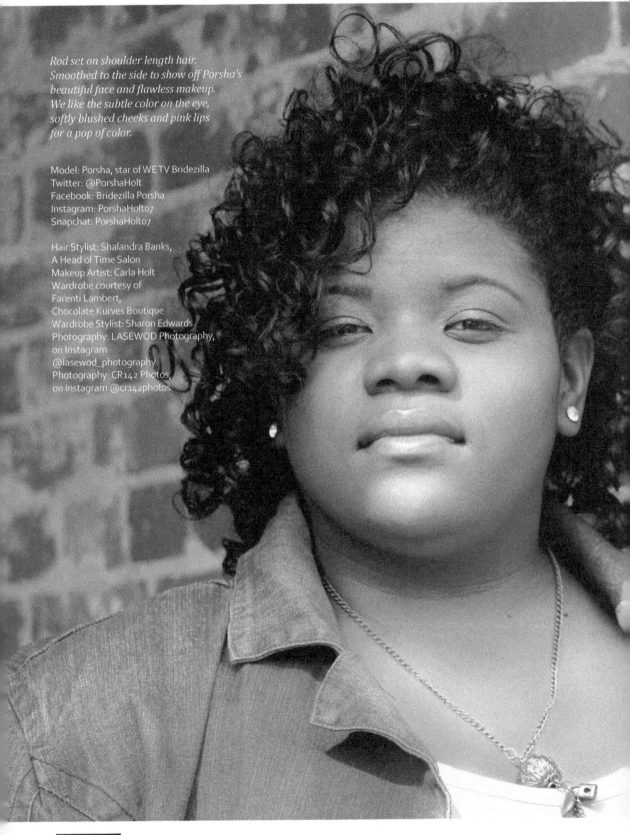

Rod set on shoulder length hair.
Smoothed to the side to show off Porsha's
beautiful face and flawless makeup.
We like the subtle color on the eye,
softly blushed cheeks and pink lips
for a pop of color.

Model: Porsha, star of WE TV Bridezilla
Twitter: @PorshaHolt
Facebook: Bridezilla Porsha
Instagram: PorshaHolt7
Snapchat: PorshaHolt7

Hair Stylist: Shalandra Banks,
A Head of Time Salon
Makeup Artist: Carla Holt
Wardrobe courtesy of
Farenti Lambert,
Chocolate Kurves Boutique
Wardrobe Stylist: Sharon Edwards
Photography: LASEWOD Photography,
on Instagram
@lasewod_photography
Photography: CR142 Photos,
on Instagram @cr142photos

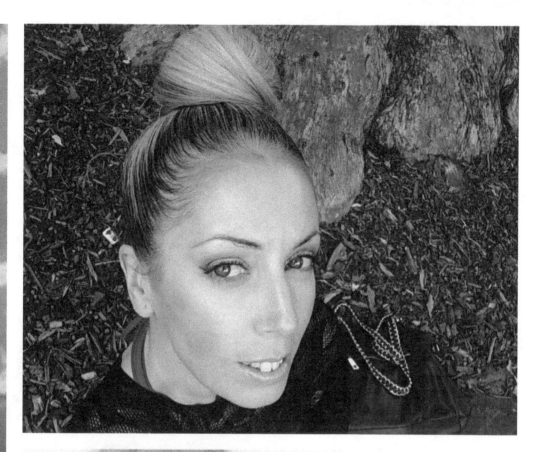

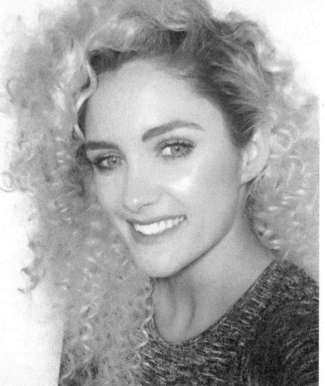

My favorite hairstyle is a top bun (top photo).

FUN FACT
I secretly still love to watch old school cartoons like Teenage Mutant Ninja Turtles and Ren & Stimpy!

Social media: Pinterest.com/ stylelifebysus | Twitter.com/ StyleBySusana | Instagram.com/ styleandlifebysusana

Favorite Styling Tool Brands:
Instyler, ghd BaByliss Curler, Andrew Barton, Lee Stafford (bottom photo)

Niamh
on Instagram @niahcullenx

STYLE NOTES
by Gabrielle

(top right) *Combing your curls out with a wide-tooth comb, will give you a more relaxed feel.*

(bottom right) *Curl your hair with a wide plate iron will give you bodyy waves that everybody loves!*

(bottom left) *Use Clip in extensions for fullness in a ponytail.*

Hair by Gabrielle Roccuzzo | Melbourne, Australia
On Instagram @_hairbygabrielle

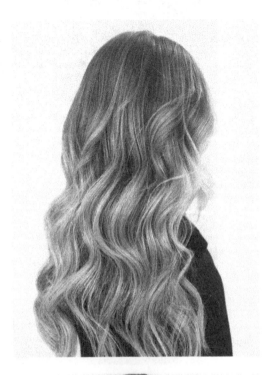

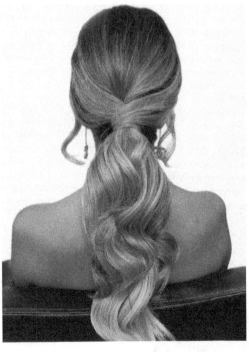

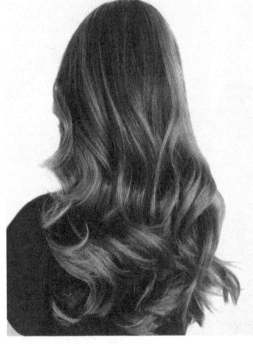

*Flip your hair upside down
and spray dry shampoo throughout
your hair for the best texture.*

Hair by Gabrielle Roccuzzo | Melbourne, Australia
On Instagram @_hairbygabrielle

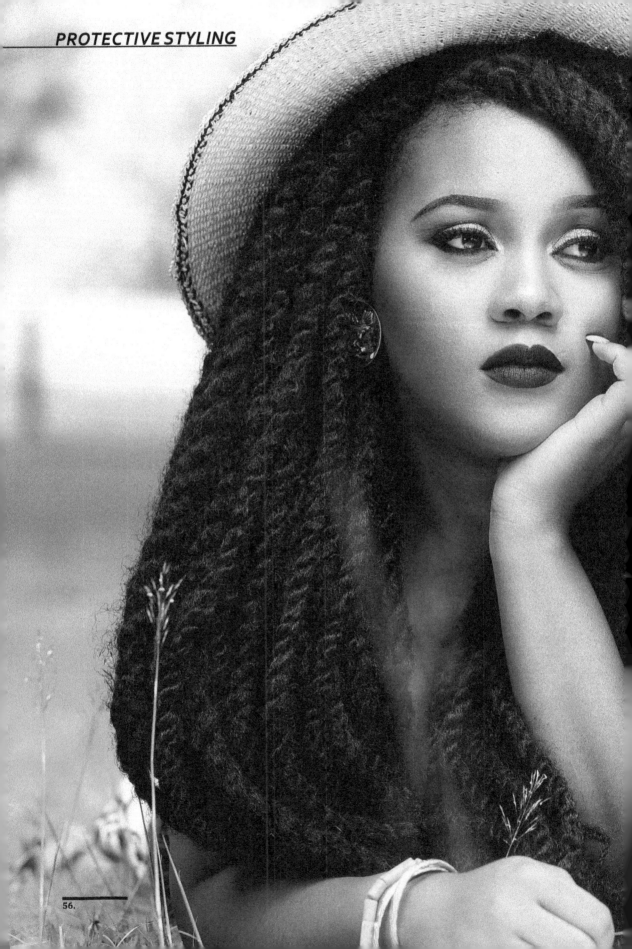

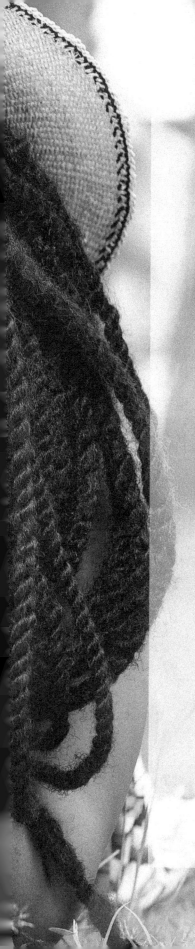

PROTECTIVE HAIRSTYLING

by Ariel Johnson

Being a natural and creating a new style everyday can get tiresome, but with protective styling your morning rituals will get a little easier. Protective styling is simple, just create a style that can hold up for a week or longer. A really popular protective style is hair extensions. Extensions comes in so many ways that there is an endless amount of style that one can come up with.

A popular extension style is braiding hair. When using braiding hair one can either style the hair individually, to the scalp, or even twisted. These styles give the natural hair time to grow without using products or heat. The braiding styles are very low maintenance and are very easy to touch up. Another favorite is hair weave extensions. Hair weave extension can be made with different textures that matches the individual's hair needs. To get a successful look, a license stylist would braid the hair to the scalp. Then with the proper needle and thread the stylist would proceed to sew the hair to the scalp braid and style as desired.

Women of all background can use a protective style on their hair. Protective styles work for women on the go, with relaxed hair, and natural hair. There are many protective styles. Some of our favorites are bantu knots, roller set curls, and of course twist outs! No matter what the occasion a protective hair style would always fit your character.

Hair Stylist & Makeup Artist:
Isoken Enofe-Asemota

EARTH DAY
by Ariel Johnson

Earth Day is an annual celebrated holiday across the globe that promotes environmental protection and awareness. That's right, thousands of rallies and outdoor projects are taken place to help keep mother Earth clean.

In 1970, the first Earth Day was celebrated. Founder Senator Gaylord Nelson of Wisconsin first created the idea of Earth Day when witnessing the damages caused by the 1969 oil spill in Santa Barbara, California. Nelson's purpose was to inform society about the environment and how to provide care for Mother Earth. Then on April 22, 1970, with the help from his 85 staff members, Nelson's plan executed and reached over 20 million people across the U.S. Many universities and public communities held rallies to teach and form plans to help protect Mother Earth from any type of pollution. The urgency of Earth Day reminds people about the importance of our humanity and with each contribution we can change our planet's future.

EARTH DAY PHOTOSHOOT
We partnered with AVEDA in Buckhead-Atlanta to celebrate Earth Month. We were so excited to take on this project and of course we worked with talented hair stylists and makeup artists at AVEDA Institute to help us pull it all together. Three models with different hair textures were chosen from our casting call. The overall hair goal was to create playful, chic, and natural looks. For makeup we wanted to show that LESS really is MORE. Each look was created using AVEDA's hair products. AVEDA's products are developed with plants, seeds, nuts and flowers which is eco-friendly and great for accommodating all textures of hair. Most products can be found in your local AVEDA store or online at www.aveda.com.

Project Manager: Kanin Curtis
Creative Director: Victor Moore
Photography: www.cr142photos.com
on Instagram: @cr142photos

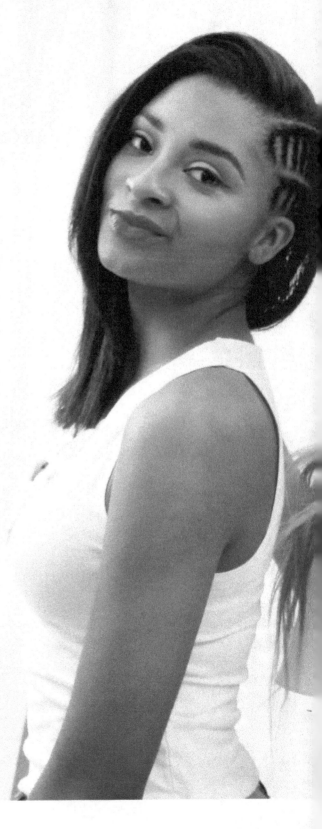

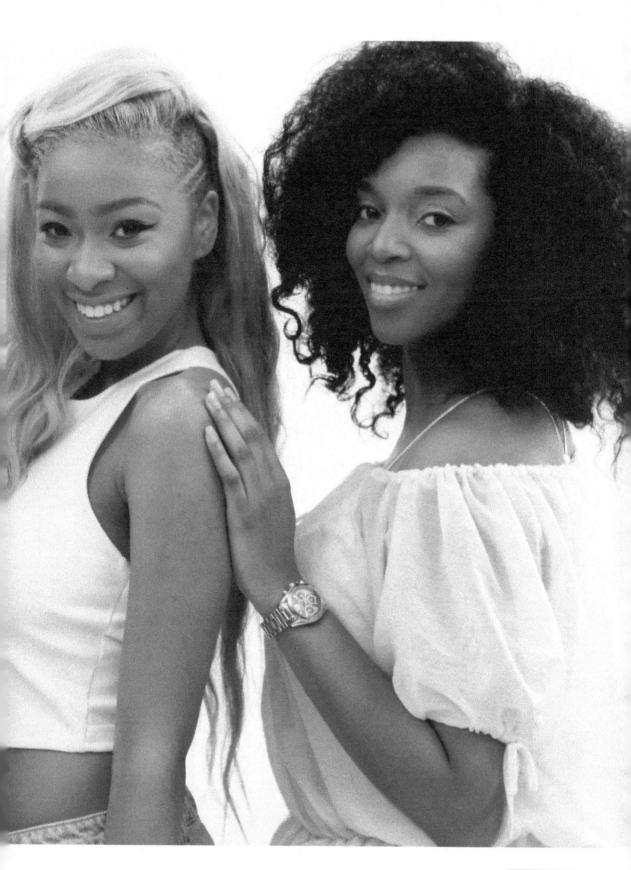

Ayana has natural hair. During her styling session, Key treated Ayana's hair using products from AVEDA's be curly line and styled her hair into three different looks. The first look has a two-strand twist on the left side that blends into a partial fro-out. The second look is a French twisted up-do. The third look (on page 61) is a textured Afro created from a twist out. Natural girls need options too and this is a great way to transform multiple looks.

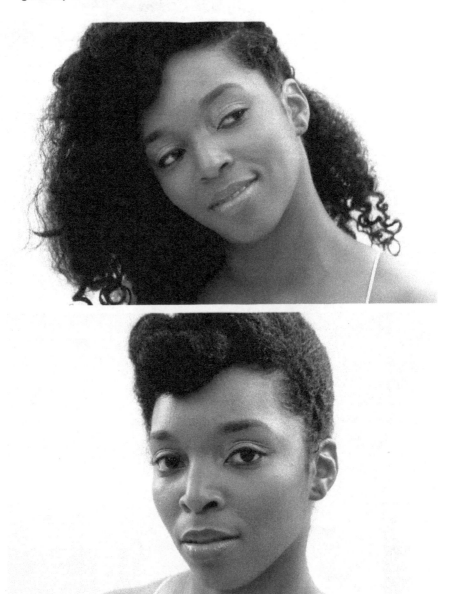

HAIR PRODUCTS
Be Curly style prep for frizz control.
Curl Controller used on the textured Afro.
To create Afro volume, we used Volumizing Spray on the roots and
sleeked Ayana's edges using Light Elements Texturizing Crème.

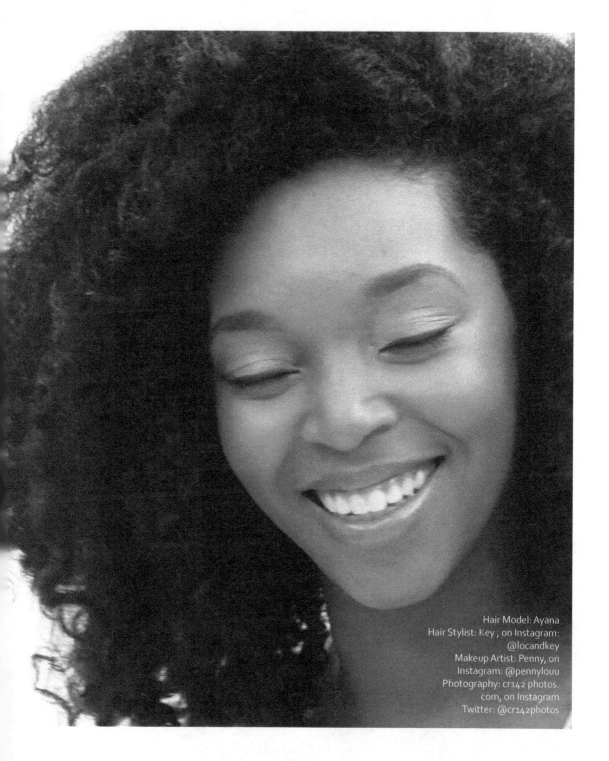

FACE

*We created an earthy look for Ayana using Mineral tinted SPF 15
moisturizer in Poplar, applied bronze, brown, yellow and green eye
shadows, Black Mosscara, Brown Eyeliner on brows. We finished her look
with a natural looking lip using Nourish-mint Agave Nectar lip glaze.*

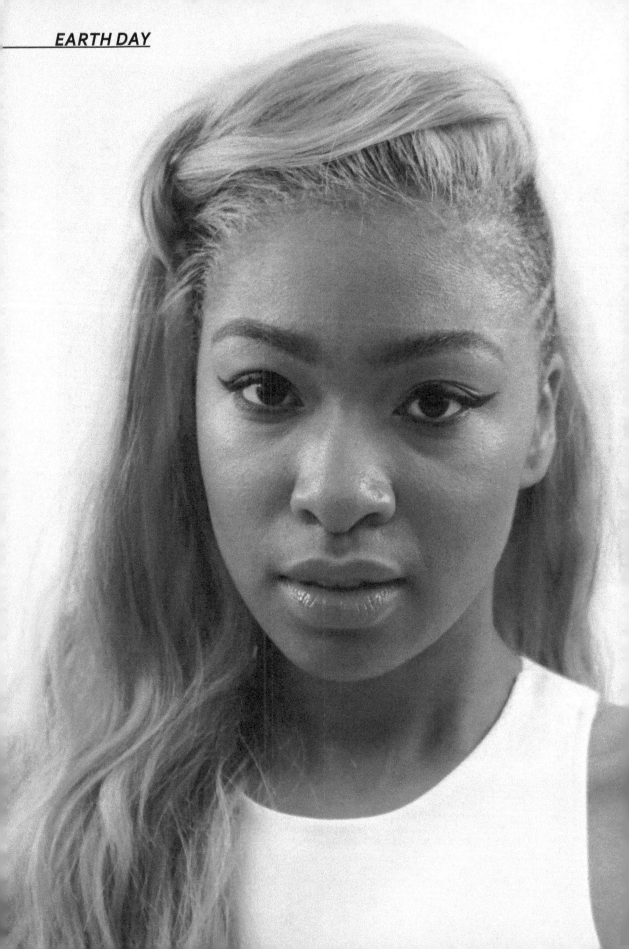

Do blondes have more fun? Probably so. Carly is sure to turn heads rocking a bleached blonde look. She has natural hair with a vixen sew-in and shaved sides. Sloan started with twisting Carly's extensions then applying heat at 400 degrees. The heat helped to settle in texture giving her a wavy look. The front right of her hair is a loose, partial plait. Sloan shaved the left side to give Carly a rocker look (see page 62). To create a second look, simply part her hair down the middle and comb the top left hair over the shaved side (see photo below).

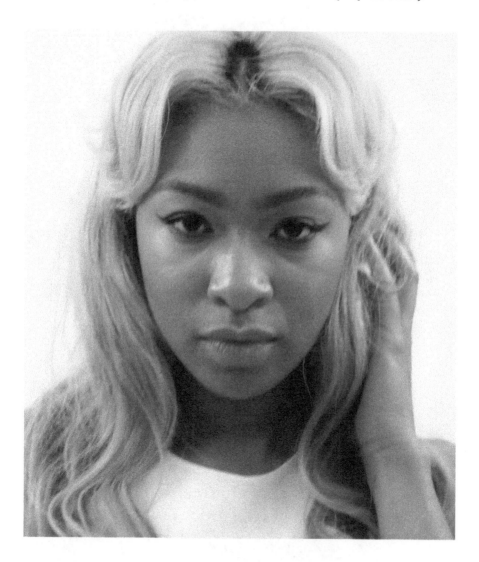

HAIR TOOLS & PRODUCTS
Nalu Waver on 400 degree setting
Air Control force for medium hold
Carly used BW by Clairol in Bleached Blonde. Use caution when bleaching your hair at home. Consult with a professional.

Model: Carly | Hair Stylist: Sloan, on Instagram: @createdbysloan
Makeup Artist: Penny, on Instagram: @pennylouu
Photography: cr142 photos.com | Instagram – Twitter: @cr142photos

Janis is transitioning from relaxed hair back to natural. This stage can be difficult because of breakage, dryness and working with two textures. We gave her a hobo chic style complimentary with dual side braids on one side and a sleek sexy look on the other (see look 1). This hairstyle can easily transform into a playful, messy look (see look 2).

LOOK 1

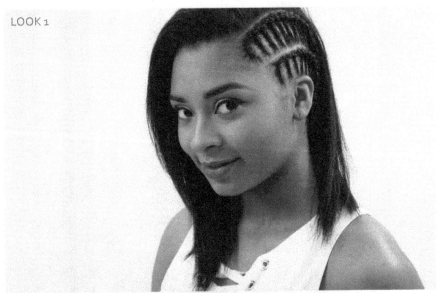

LOOK 2

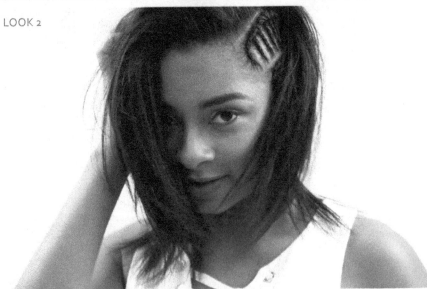

HAIR PRODUCTS

Caution should be used when using flatirons. Ensure that to use the right temperature for your hair type. First, we applied Smooth Infusion Naturally Straight to achieve a straighter look. We used a ½ inch flat iron on 300 degrees on Janis' hair then smoothed her edges using Control Paste with flax seed for total edge control.

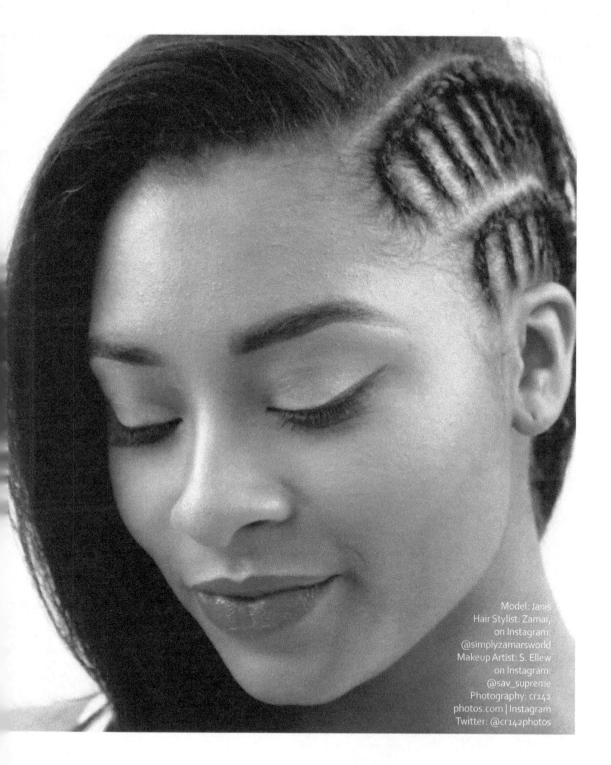

Model: Janis
Hair Stylist: Zamar,
on Instagram:
@simplyzamarsworld
Makeup Artist: S. Ellew
on Instagram:
@sav_supreme
Photography: cr142
photos.com | Instagram
Twitter: @cr142photos

FACE

We created a custom color for Janis using Mineral tinted SPF 15 moisturizer mixed with Popular and Bark then applied a concoction of Almond, Ginger, and Carob Foundation Powder. A light layer of concealer was applied in Inner Light Peace and Nutmeg. Rose Blossom on her cheeks for a soft blush effect and a hint of color on her eyes using Spark Eye Shadow. To finish off the look, we used Black Orchid Eye Definer and Black Mosscara to refine her eyes. Eye Definer in Cacao and Snap Dragon on lips.

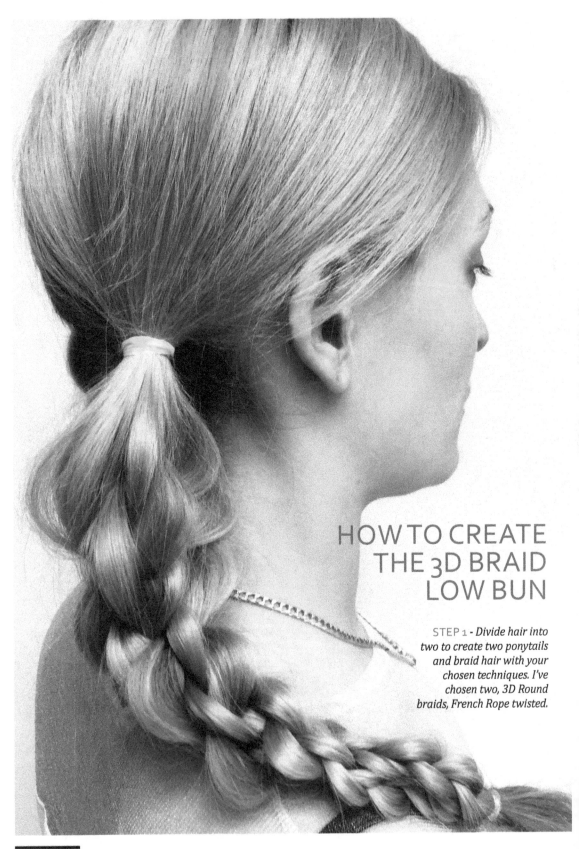

HOW TO CREATE THE 3D BRAID LOW BUN

STEP 1 - *Divide hair into two to create two ponytails and braid hair with your chosen techniques. I've chosen two, 3D Round braids, French Rope twisted.*

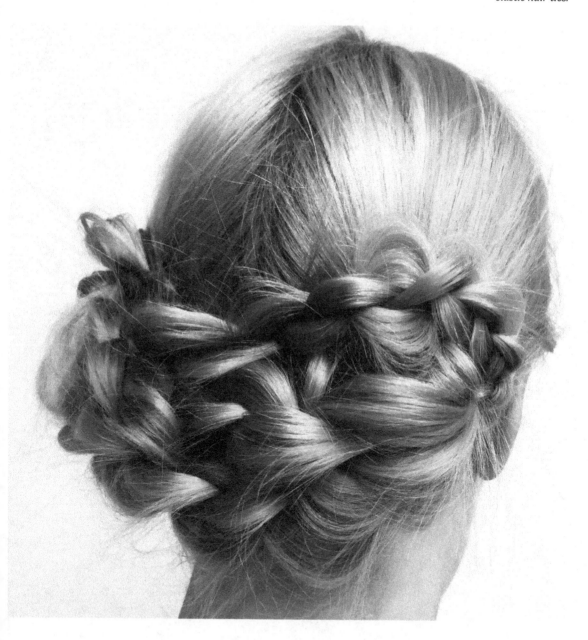

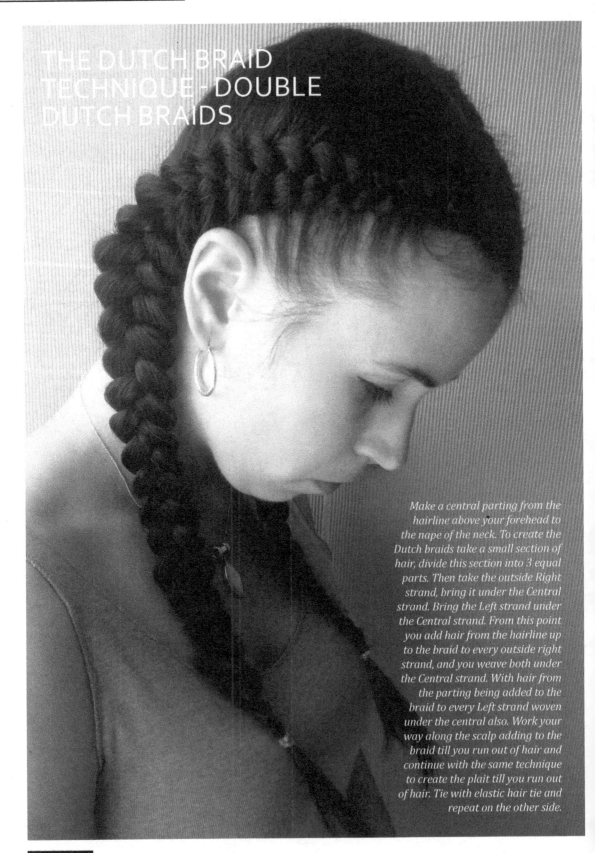

THE DUTCH BRAID TECHNIQUE - DOUBLE DUTCH BRAIDS

Make a central parting from the hairline above your forehead to the nape of the neck. To create the Dutch braids take a small section of hair, divide this section into 3 equal parts. Then take the outside Right strand, bring it under the Central strand. Bring the Left strand under the Central strand. From this point you add hair from the hairline up to the braid to every outside right strand, and you weave both under the Central strand. With hair from the parting being added to the braid to every Left strand woven under the central also. Work your way along the scalp adding to the braid till you run out of hair and continue with the same technique to create the plait till you run out of hair. Tie with elastic hair tie and repeat on the other side.

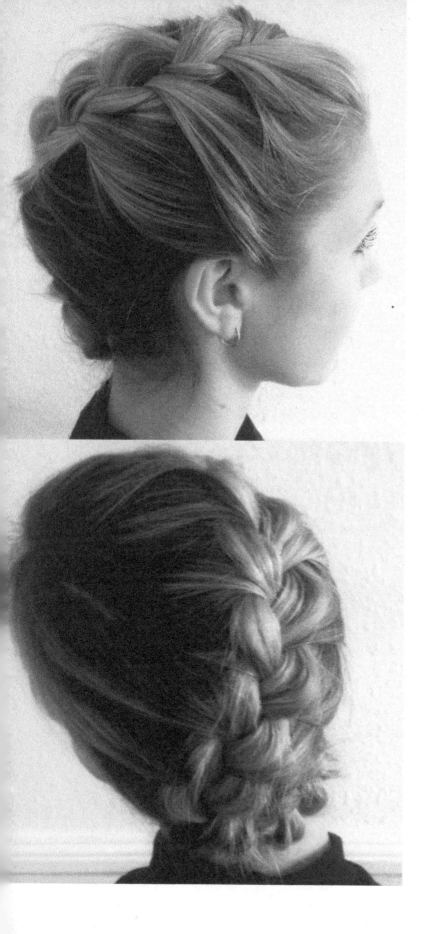

THE FRENCH BRAID TECHNIQUE

To create the French braids take a small section of hair, divide this section into 3 equal parts. Then take the outside Right strand, bring it over the Central strand. Bring the Left strand over the Central strand. From this point add hair from the hairline to the braid to every outside Right and Left strand you weave, braiding both over the Central strand. Keep working along your scalp adding hair to the braid till you run out and continue with the same technique to create the plait till you run out of hair. Tie with elastic hair tie and pancake to create a looser more casual look.

Braid Collection presented by
Joel Benjamin,
on Instagram @hairbyjoel
Hairstylist & Director
at HairbyJoël
HairbyJoel.co.uk

Printed in June 2019
by Rotomail Italia S.p.A., Vignate (MI) - Italy